Gheranda Samhita

Ashwini Kumar Aggarwal

जय गुरुदेव

ISBN13: 978-81-947338-7-4 Paperback Edition
ISBN13: 978-81-947338-3-6 Hardbound Edition
ISBN13: 978-81-947338-2-9 Digital Edition
ISBN13: 978-81-950348-4-0 B/W Low Price Edition

Title: Gheranda Samhita the foundation of Modern Yoga

Printed and Published by
Devotees of Sri Sri Ravi Shankar Ashram
34 Sunny Enclave, Devigarh Road,
Patiala 147001, Punjab, India

https://advaita56.weebly.com/
The Art of Living Centre

https://www.artofliving.org/

12th August 2020 Krishna Janmashtami, Bhadrapada Ashtami Budhavasara, Krishna Paksha, Rohini Nakshatra, Varsha Ritu Vikram Samvat 2077 Pramadi, Saka Era 1942 Sharvari

1st Edition August 2020

जय गुरुदेव

Dedication

Sri Sri Ravi Shankar

who revealed to us the powerful breathing technique known as the
Sudarshan Kriya

an offering at thy lotus feet

Acknowledgements

An impeccable inspiration by Jagjit Singh Grewal who follows morning Sadhana and Sudarshan Kriya since 29 January 2009 without a break with a 12-year commitment till 29 January 2021.

Content Creation Design Credits

Dipanshu Aggarwal   Apurav Gupta
Himika Sharma   Radhika Aggarwal

Dipanshu17June2020 Shirsasana
https://www.youtube.com/watch?v=YpxstzvldQw

EEG signal-based classification before and after combined Yoga and Sudarshan Kriya
https://www.sciencedirect.com/science/article/abs/pii/S03043940
19303738

Front Cover Image Credits

Gurudev's Guidance painting by A. Manivelu
https://www.himalayanacademy.com/view/manivelu-5-kutumba-
sadhanas-following-preceptor

Blessing

Intellectually we know everything. But when the moment comes, when the negativity comes like a flood, it just overpowers you. Right? It just throws you off all the knowledge you have heard, read, and understood…No? Anger comes, jealousy comes, fear comes.

What to do?
Here Breathing techniques, Meditation, Sudarshan Kriya.

Kriya helps in a great manner. In an unbelievable fashion it helps you overcome the flood of emotions. Once we learn Kriya, it's like a mechanism within you, automatically there is a valve in you that functions. It helps you overcome negative emotions…much easily.
https://www.youtube.com/watch?v=A27L9oknmic

A study done at Yale found that by practicing SKY (Sudarshan Kriya), students reported improvements in six areas of well-being: depression, stress, mental health, mindfulness, positive affect, and social connectedness. @SriSri

Sri Sri Ravi Shankar
Bangalore Ashram, Jul 28, 2020

https://www.srisriravishankar.org/sudarshan-kriya
https://www.ncbi.nlm.nih.gov/pmc/articles/PMC3573542/

Prayer

ॐ भद्रं कर्णेभिः शृणुयाम देवाः । भद्रं पश्ये माक्षभिर् यजत्राः ।
स्थिरैरङ्गैस् तुष्टुवा(गुं)सस्तनूभिः । व्यशेम देवहितं यदायुः ॥
स्वस्ति न इन्द्रो वृद्धश्रवाः । स्वस्ति नः पूषा विश्ववेदाः ।
स्वस्ति नस्ताक्ष्यो अरिष्टनेमिः । स्वस्ति नो बृहस्पतिर्दधातु ॥
ॐ शान्तिः शान्तिः शान्तिः ॥

oṃ bhadraṃ karṇebhiḥ śṛṇuyāma devāḥ | bhadraṃ paśye

mākṣabhir yajatrāḥ | sthirairaṅgais tuṣṭuvā(gum)sastanūbhiḥ |

vyaśema devahitaṃ yadāyuḥ ‖ svasti na indro vṛddhaśravāḥ |

svasti naḥ pūṣā viśvavedāḥ | svasti nastārkṣyo ariṣṭanemiḥ |

svasti no bṛhaspatirdadhātu ‖

oṃ śāntiḥ śāntiḥ śāntiḥ ‖

O Divine Light!
May our ears listen to the sacred and the auspicious.
May our eyes see the propitious allowing us
To come together to partake of wisdom.

May our limbs be firm and body attuned to long endurances.
May our senses function with full alertness and
May the sense of contentment be strong.

May our good thoughts form a discus to shield us and
May our education give us a shining personality.

Peace in our heart, in our body and in our environs.

http://vedicheritage.gov.in/Taittiriya_Aranyaka/KYTA_1.mp4

Bhagavad Gita

युक्ताहारविहारस्य , युक्तचेष्टस्य कर्मसु ।
युक्तस्वप्नावबोधस्य , योगो भवति दुःखहा ॥ ६.१७

yuktaahaaravihaarasya, yuktace.s.tasya karmasu ।

yuktasvapnaavabodhasya, yogo bhavati du.hkhahaa ॥ 6.17

6.17 Be regulated in food and exercise; be balanced in activity and duty. Take proper sleep and rest, and nurture senses equitably. Such a lifestyle leads to freedom from pain. It frees one from suffering. It extinguishes the pangs of remorse and banishes turmoil from life.

Regulated food includes eating fresh, vegetarian, timely meals. Regulated exercise includes Yogasana, walking, swimming, sports or gymnasium in a proper environment.

Balance in activity and duty includes having good teamwork, using the right tools, maintaining good posture and taking sufficient breaks for rest and hobby. Proper sleep includes using correct cot and mattress and sleeping with the lights off.

Nurturing senses equitably includes paying attention to brushing twice daily, taking care of hair and skin by appropriate massage, taking care of eyes and ears and ensuring correct breathing.

Etymology of word YOGA in Sanskrit

There are 3 roots in the Dhatupatha of Panini.

1177 युज समाधौ । चित्तवृत्तिनिरोधे । meditate, do upasana, concentrate 4c 71 युज़ँ । युज् । युज्यते । A । अनिट् । अ० ।

1806 युज संयमने । आधृषीयः । वैकल्पिकः णिचः । restrain, check, discipline, concentrate 10c 273 युज़ँ । युज् । योजयति / ते, योजति । U । सेट् । स० । योजि । योजय ।

1444 युजिर् योगे । join, unite, become one, be ready. *Famous words* योगः , योगी , युक्तः । 7c 7 युजिँर् । युज् । युनक्ति / युङ्क्ते । U । अनिट् । स० । युक्तः युक्ता युक्तम् । युक्तवान् युक्तवती युक्तवत् ।

Contents

CHAPTER 2 – ASANA – THIRTY TWO TYPES OF BODY POSTURES   57

Classical Yogasana Texts

The Advaita Vedanta tradition is all about achieving Yoga. Here Yoga is used in the sense of uniting with the Pure Self, to become well integrated in the functioning of body, mind, speech, and heart.

There are many ancient and classical texts that highlight
- Asanas or Body Postures
- Pranayama or Breath Control techniques, and
- Meditation and Contemplation processes

to achieve this oneness easily and with long-term stability. These are the **Hatha Yoga or Raja Yoga texts**, which means being earnestly committed to **Body and Mind Disciplines**.

Principal among these are:
- Yoga Vasistha
- Bhagavad Gita
- Patanjali Yoga Sutras
- Thirumoolar Mandiram of Tamil Sage Thirumoolar
- Yoga Taravali of Adi Shankaracharya
- Yoga Yajnavalkya Samhita, 2nd century BC - Sage Yajnavalka
- Goraksha Shatakam, circa 10th century AD of Gorakshanatha
- Vasistha Samhita: Chapter on Yoga, circa 1300 AD
- Hatha Yoga Pradipika circa 1350 AD by Svatmarama
- HathaRatnavali circa 1650 AD by Srinivasa Bhatta
- Gheranda Samhita circa 1750 AD of Gheranda Muni
- Joga Pradipika of Jayatarama, circa 1800 AD
- Shiva Samhita

Preface

Out of all the texts that enumerate various Asana and Pranayama and Meditation, the one that explains body postures and breath control with crystal clear clarity is the Gheranda Samhita.

Gheranda Samhita is also known as **Ghata Samhita** which means "Health & Fitness through stretching and molding the **clay pot** like anatomical Body in different ways".

Gheranda = name of a Sage
Samhita = proper collection of his Teaching
Ghata = clay pot = anatomical body

The text is called saptanga or seven limbed, and closely models the eight limbed ashtanga of Patanjali Yoga Sutras. Also notice that Goraksha Shatakam teaches the same in six limbed shatanga, while Hatha Yoga Pradipika discusses it in four chapters chaturanga.

Gheranda Samhita is in the form of a dialogue between
- Gheranda Muni the preceptor and
- Chandakapali the pupil

Here we give a factual description of the Asanas and Breathing techniques as popularly practiced today and relevant for the common man who is seeking to learn Yoga for his betterment, upliftment and overall success in life.

It goes without saying that these are advanced techniques, and must be learnt from a living Master or in a school having a tradition of teaching Yoga. It is quite impossible to comprehend the matter just by reading it or seeing it on TV. This text is to aid those who have learnt it the proper way already.

The 84 Asanas commonly practiced

All the Hatha Yoga texts mention 84 lakh asanas, and the Gheranda Samhita says that 84 are commonly learnt in all schools of Yoga. The word "lakh" is used here in the sense of variations according to different body types and climates and not to mean a number.

In different Yoga Schools, the Yoga Acharyas teach around 84 asanas to their students, as they build up the flexibility and strength of their wards. These 84 asanas are not fixed, each school shall have a slightly different set. Hence the usage of the word "lakh" in the ancient texts.

Yogic practice and discipline are for aligning our emotions and integrating our behaviour to the highest standards of society. This involves tuning the various energy centers in the aural body and the poses and breathing and meditation taught helps to achieve a very difficult target – overall success with good health and integrity.

The number 84 = 7 Chakras x 12 Poses for each energy center, where 12 are the constellations that specify the journey of the planets as depicted in the Jyotisha diamond matrix chart. These 7 chakras and 12 moods & temperaments combine to give the number 84, and that is emphasized in each text as the number of postures one must learn.

Different schools teach a variant set of postures. The aim is to cover the whole anatomy. The Gheranda Samhita further goes on to describe 32 asanas in detail, with a note that only 32 out of the 84 are ultimately to be practiced on a regular basis. As we also see in our daily practice, Surya Namaskar has 12 poses and Padmasadhana has 20, so the total becomes 32, which is a set to be practiced daily.

We all can take the following five courses to experience the Yoga in totality and make it personal.

1. The Art of Living Happiness Course (HP)
   https://www.artofliving.org/happiness-program
2. The Art of Living Advanced Meditation Course (AMC)
   https://www.artofliving.org/art-silence-retreat
3. The Art of Living Do Something Now Course (DSN)
   https://www.artofliving.org/other-graduate-programs
4. The Art of Living Sahaj Samadhi Course (SS)
   https://www.artofliving.org/sahaj-samadhi-meditation
5. The Art of Living Sri Sri Yoga Course (SSY)
   https://www.artofliving.org/yoga

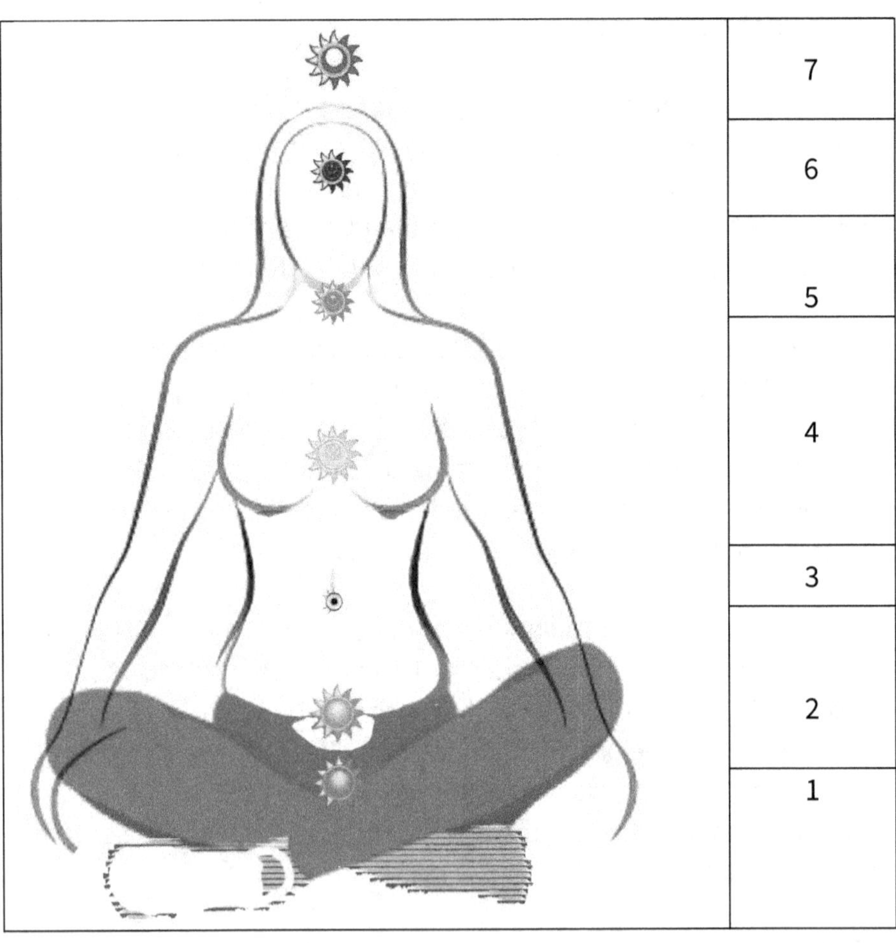

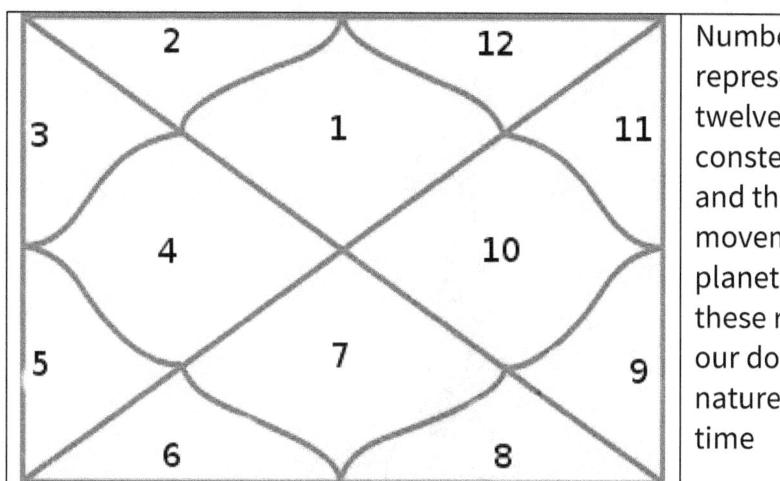

Numbers represent the twelve constellations, and the movement of planets in these represent our dominant nature at that time

The asanas which we learn in our Yoga school are of two types, dynamic and static, and we mix these in our practice:

1. Prayer Namaste = pranaamasana

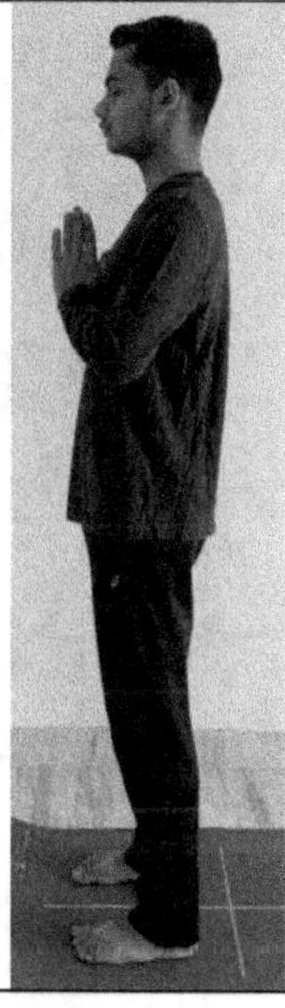

2. Up and Back = uttanahastasana	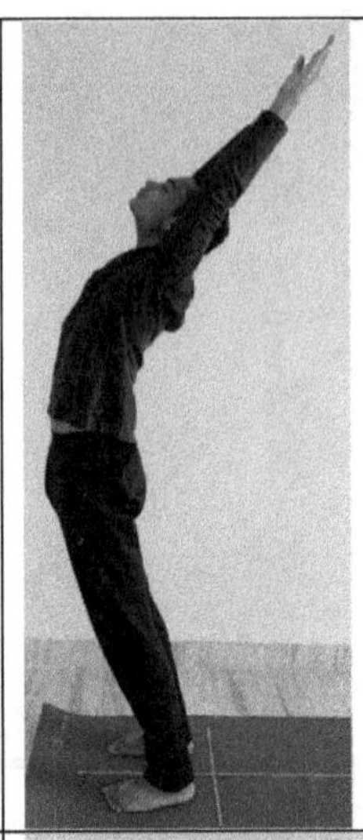
3. Forward and down = padahastasana	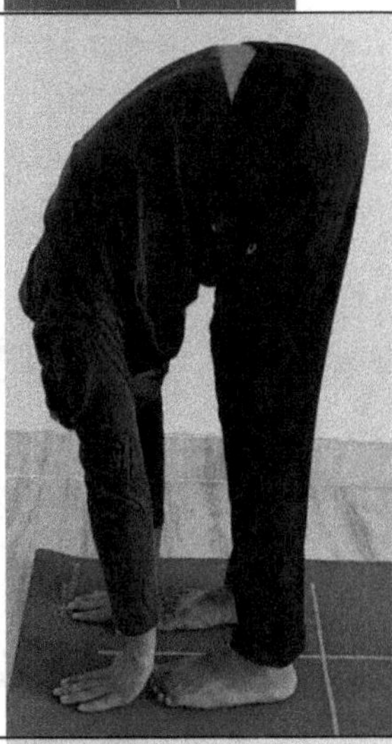
4. Equestrian = ashvasanchalanasana (similar asana with alternate leg in front)	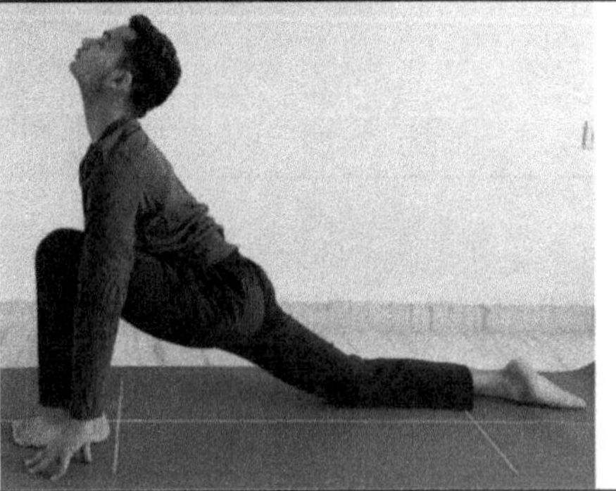

5.	Plank = caturanga dandasana	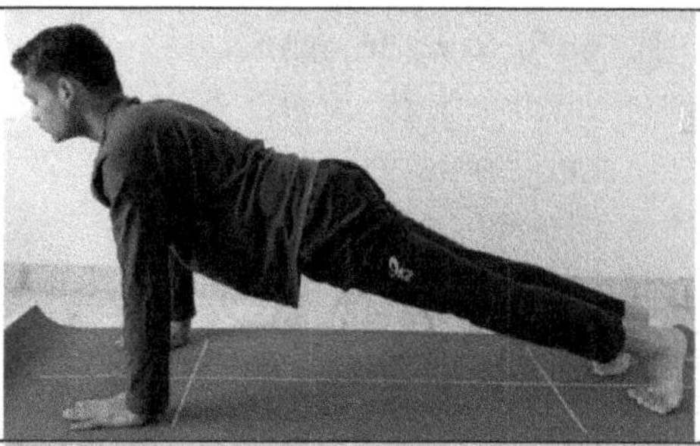
6.	Slide to bow down = ashtangapranaam	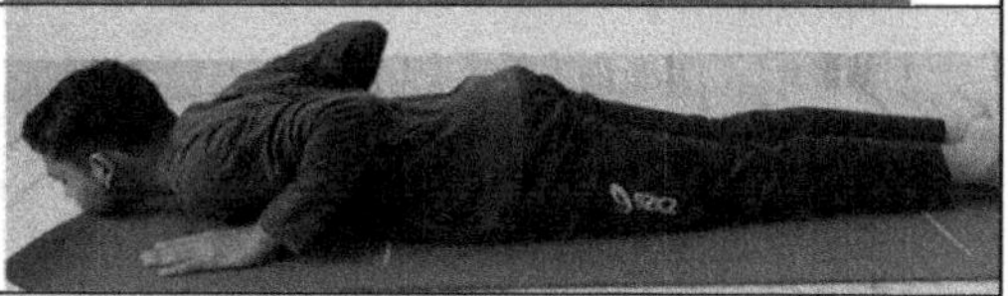
7.	Cobra = bhujangasana	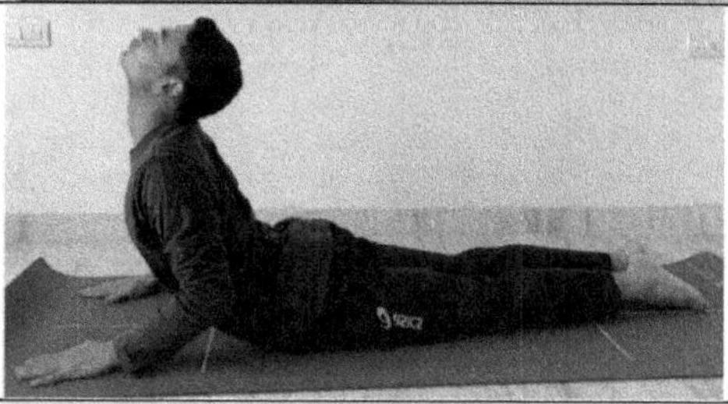
8.	Mountain = adhomukha svanasana	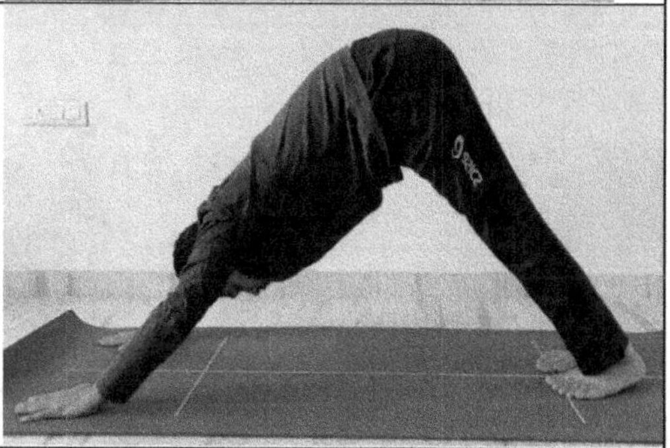
9.	Corpse = shavasana	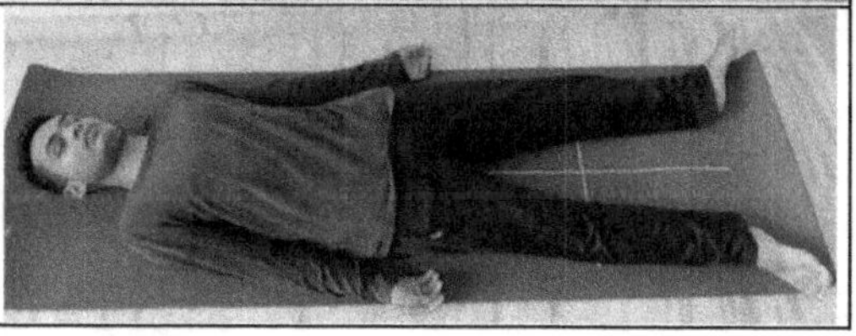

10. Lotus = padmasana (ardha padmasana can be done with alternate leg also)	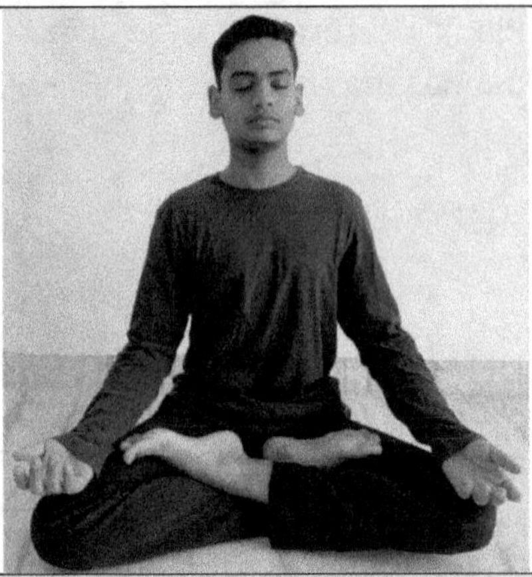
11. Body rotation	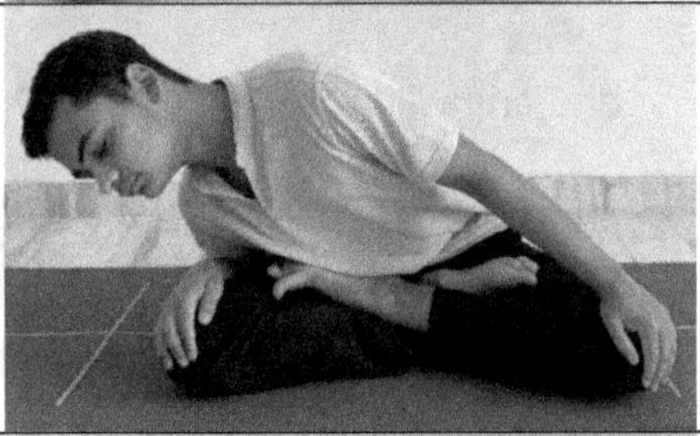
12. Locust = shalabhasana (alternate legs and both legs)	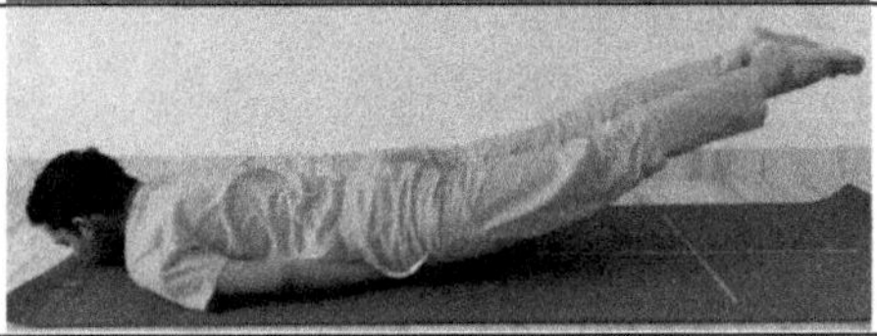
13. Superman = Viparit Shalabhasana	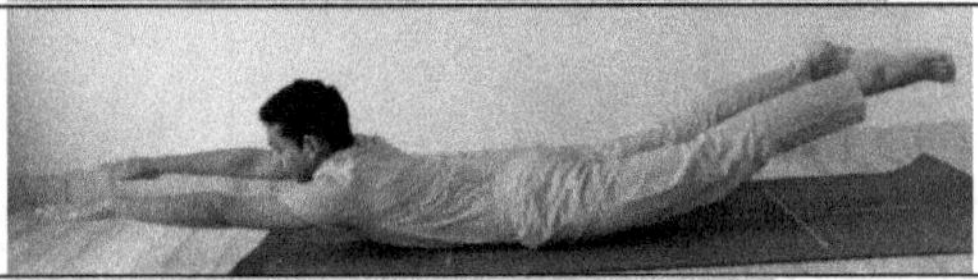
14. Bow = dhanurasana	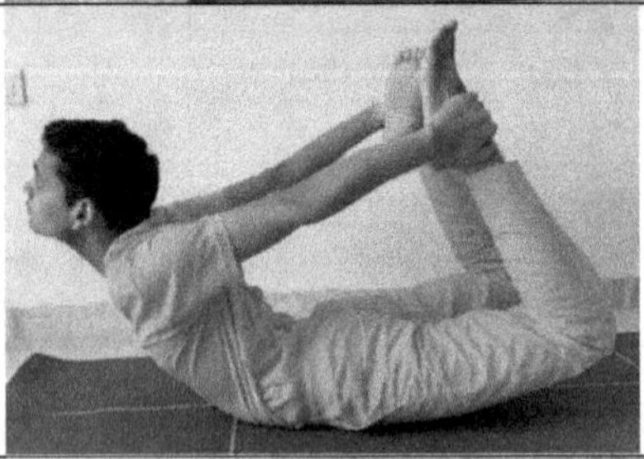
15. Crocodile = makarasana	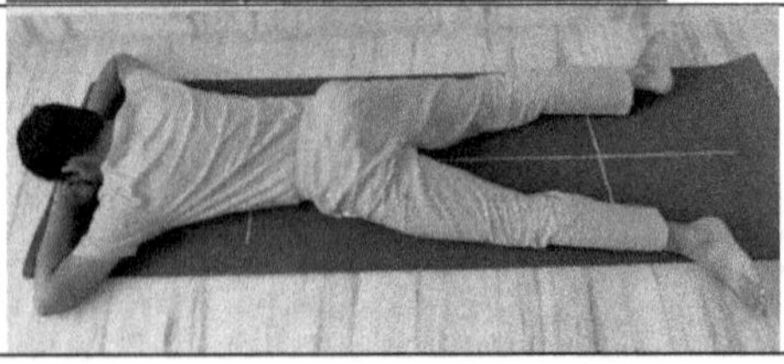

16. Lying down on side = suptavishnuasana (similar asana with alternate leg position)	
17. Boat = naukasana	
18. Wind release = pavanmuktasana (with alternate legs and both legs)	
19. Shoulder stand = sarvangasana	
20. Plough = halasana	

21. Fish = matsyasana	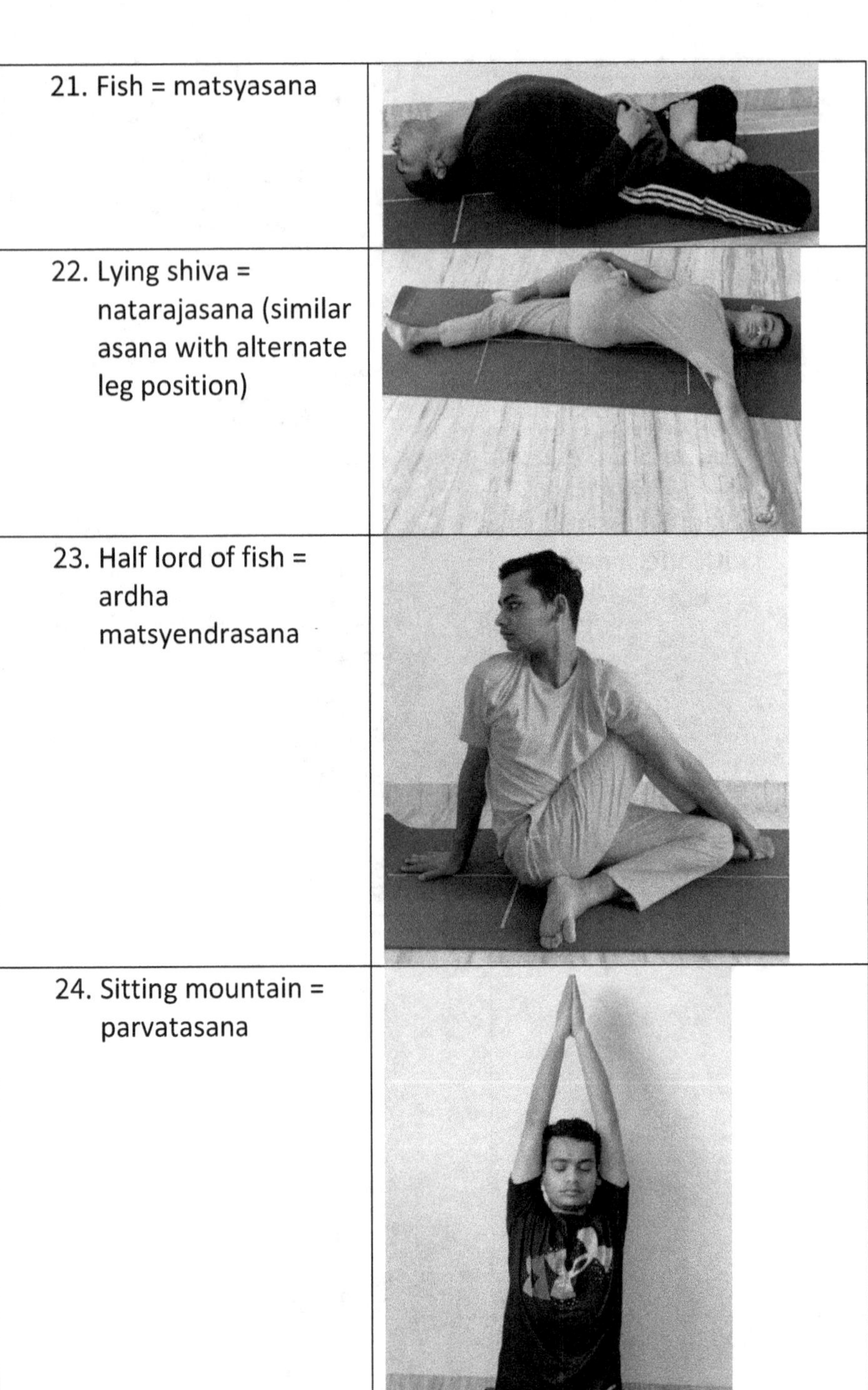
22. Lying shiva = natarajasana (similar asana with alternate leg position)	
23. Half lord of fish = ardha matsyendrasana	
24. Sitting mountain = parvatasana	

25. Child = yogamudra	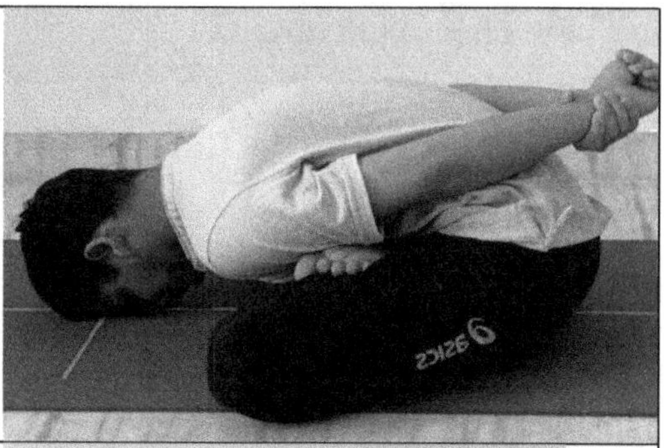
26. Rabbit = shashankasana	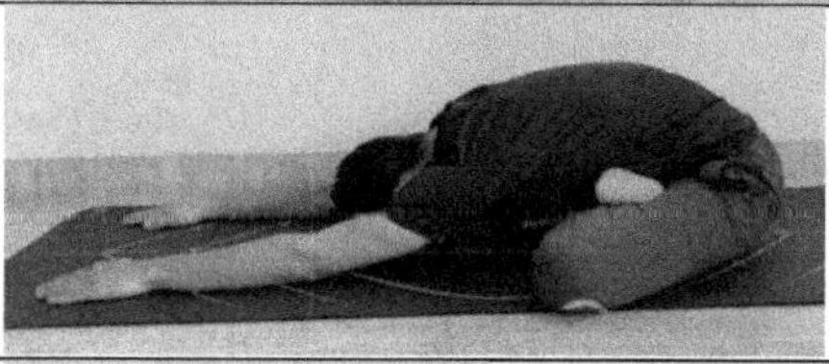
27. Superbrain yoga =	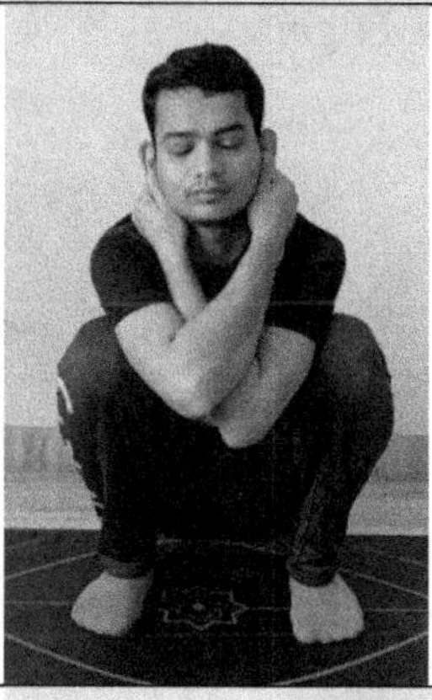
28. Power walk	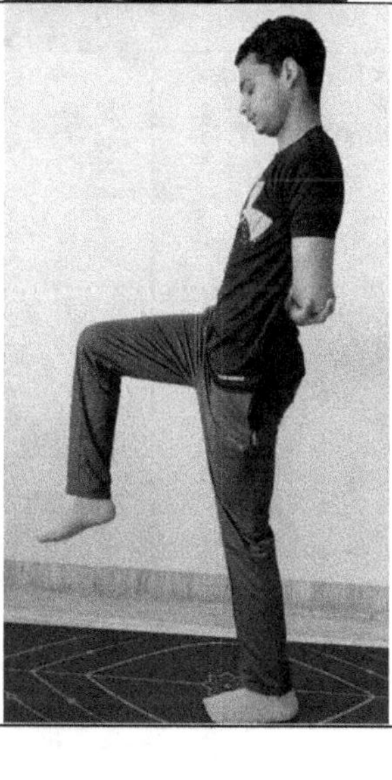

29. Chair = utkatasana	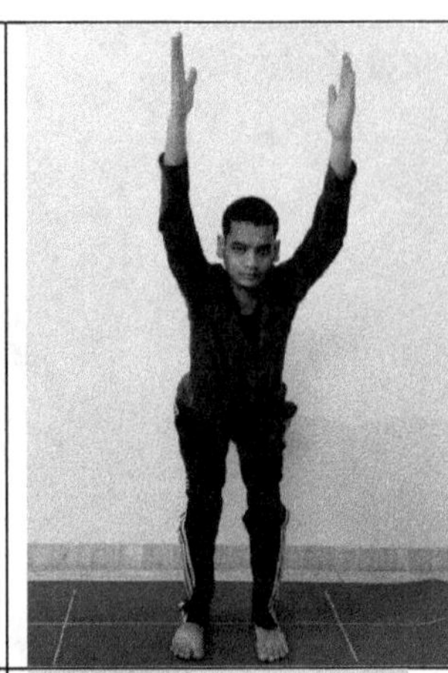
30. Joint rotation – neck, shoulder, waist, knee, ankle, fingers, wrist, palms	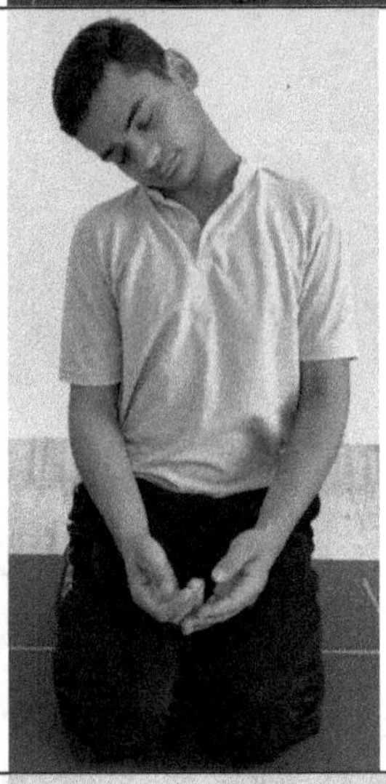
31. Dancing Shiva = natarajasana	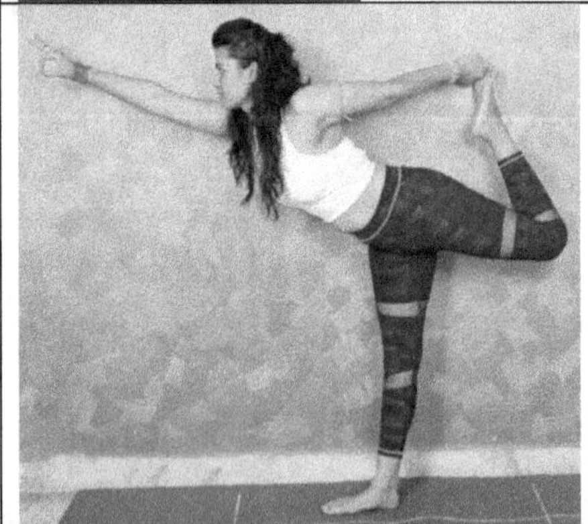

32. Standing tall = tadasana	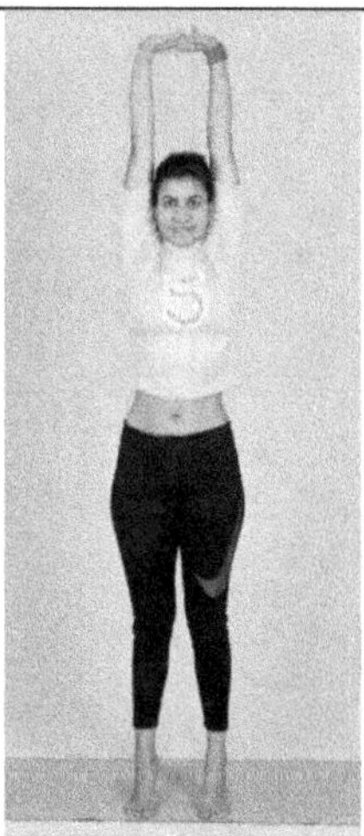
33. Warrior1 = virabhadrasana	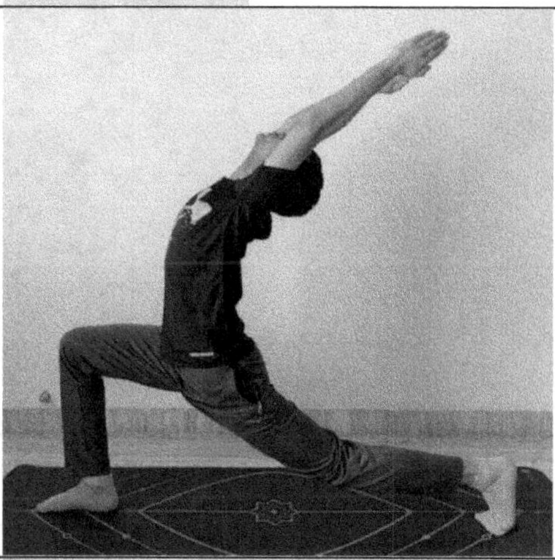
34. Warrior2 = virabhadrasana	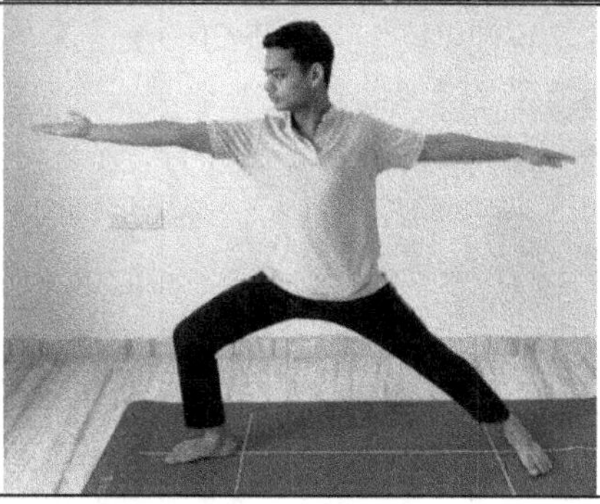

35. Warrior3 = virabhadrasana	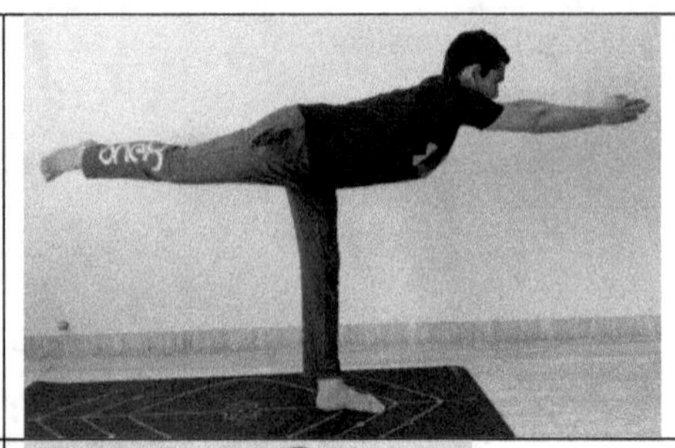
36. Tree = vrikshasana	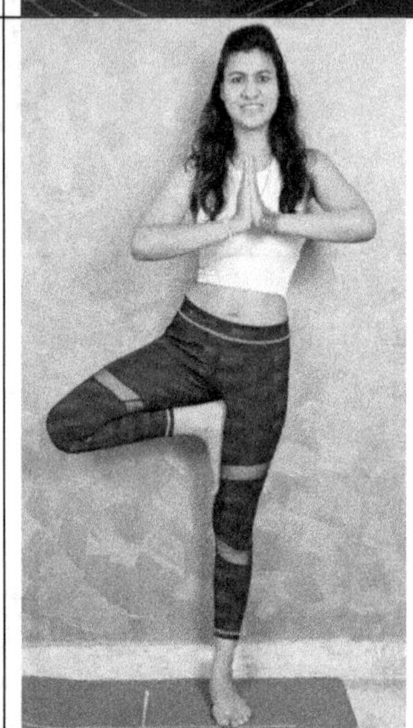
37. Swaying Tree = koneasana (tiryak tadasana - asanas on either side)	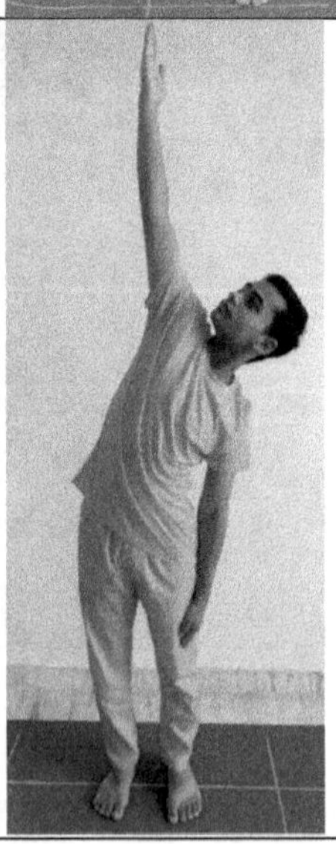

38. Two angle = dvikonasana

39. Triangle = trikonasana

40. Raised ashtanga pranaam

41. Standing spinal twist = katichakrasana	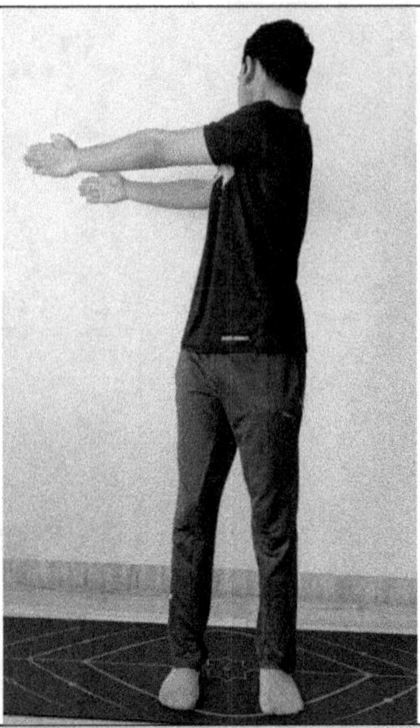
42. Pigeon = kapotasana	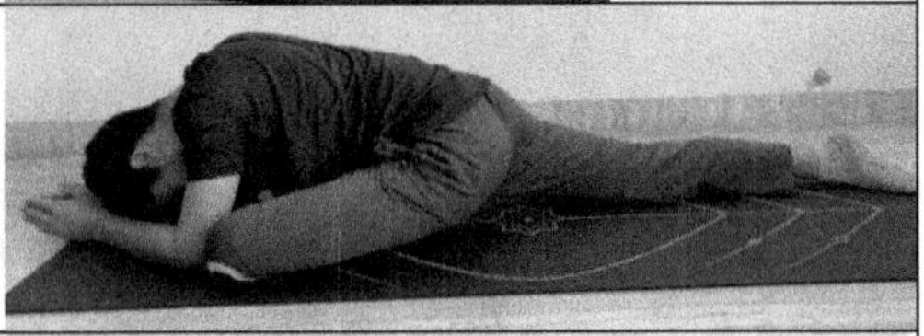
43. Raised Pigeon = uttana kapotasana	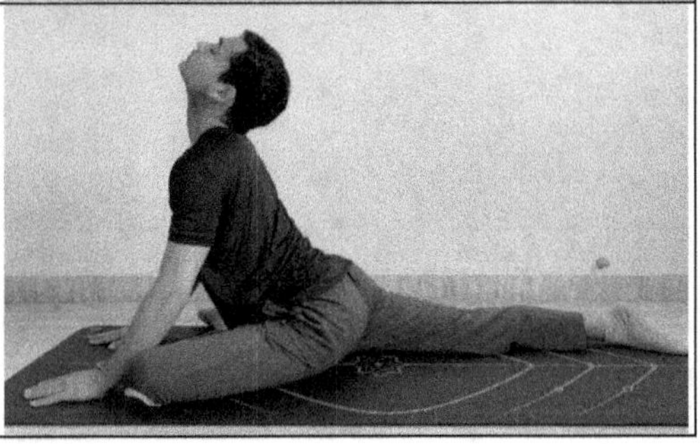

44. Potty Squat = malasana	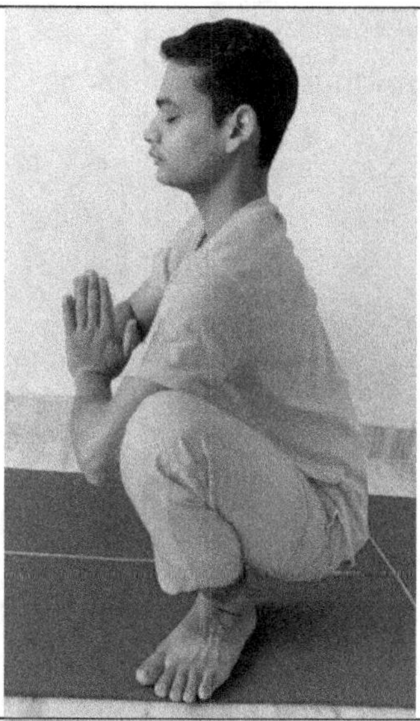
45. Eagle = garudasana	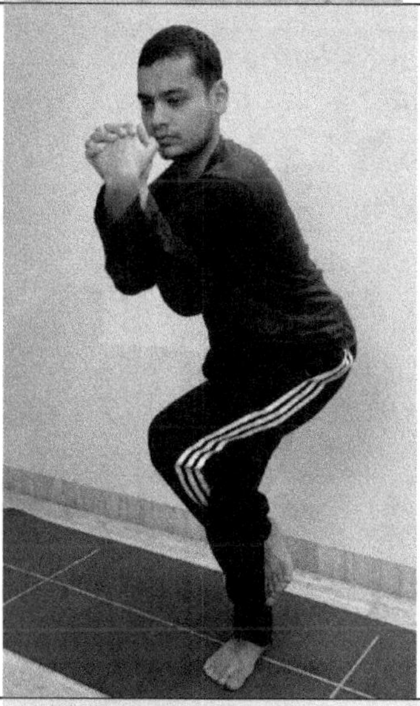
46. Wheel = ardha chakrasana	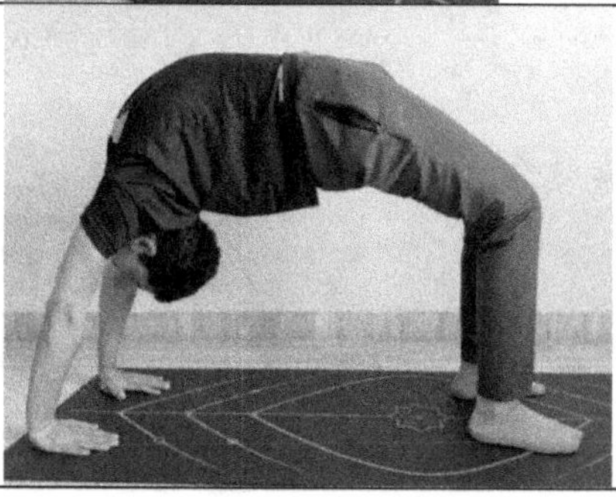

47. Bridge = setubandhasana	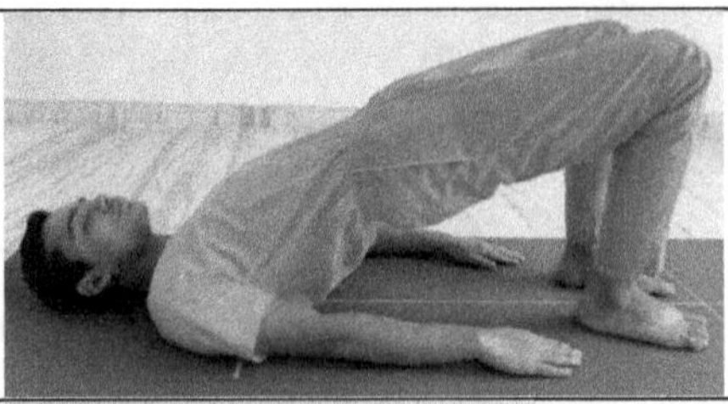
48. Camel = ushtrasana	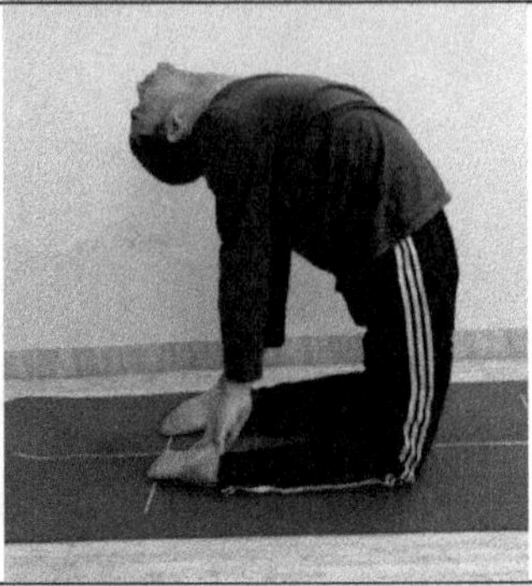
49. Serpent = Sarpasana	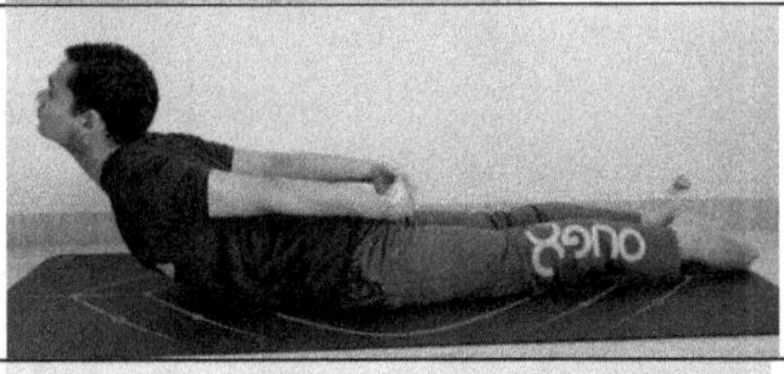
50. Legs up = Viparitakaraniasana	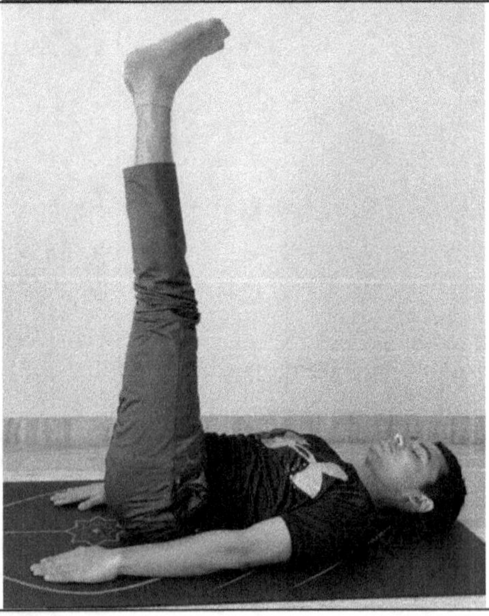

51. Upward facing Dog = Urdhva mukha svanasana	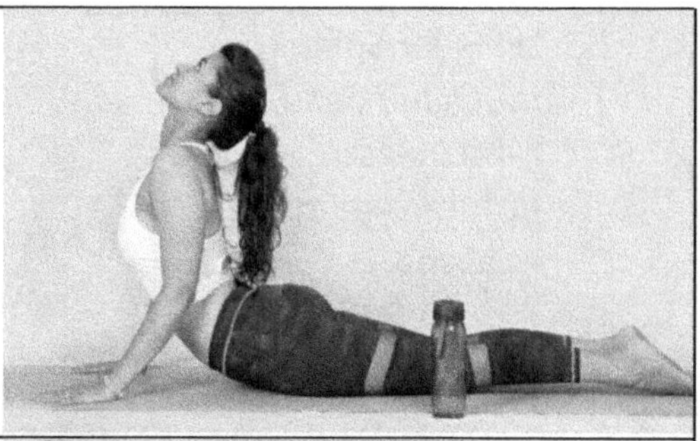
52. Cat Stretch = marjariasana (dynamic spine and head movements)	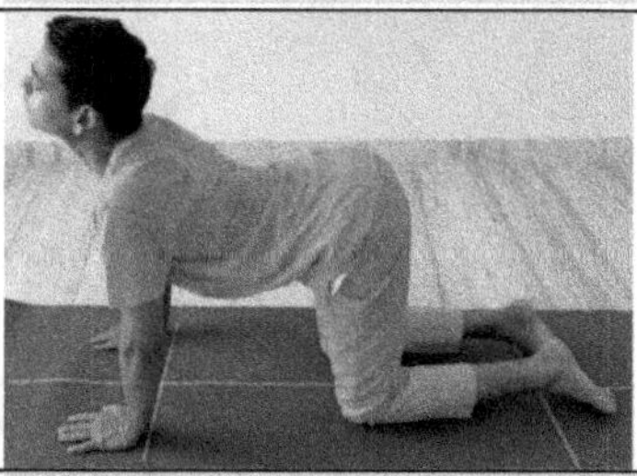
53. Cobra Twist = tiryak bhujangasana	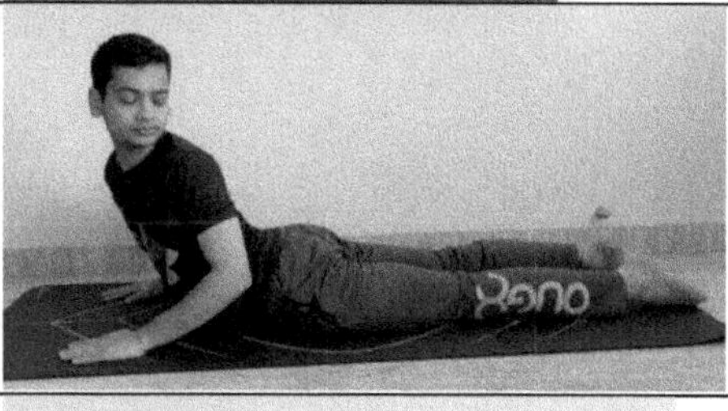
54. Raised Spine = uttana merudanda	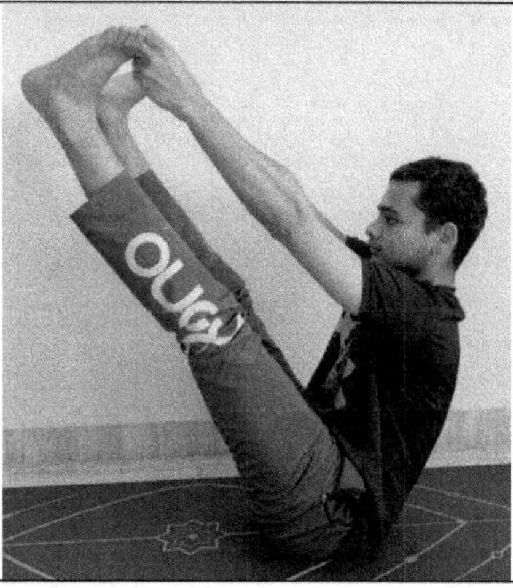

55. Lying lift Spine to touch hands to raised legs = utthitahastamerudandasana	
56. Tiger = vyaghrasana	
57. Dolphin	
58. Mill = chakkichalanasana	
59. Full Stretch lying down	

60. Crow walk = kakachalanasana	
61. Wild thing	
62. Pendulum = dolasana	

63. Lion = simhasana	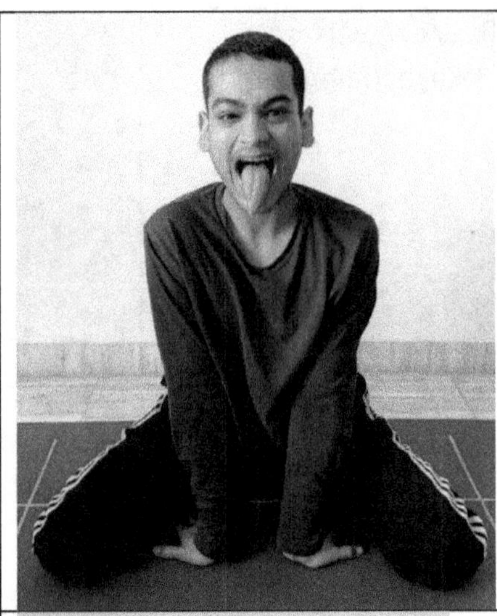
64. Sitting Head to one knee = Janusirsasana	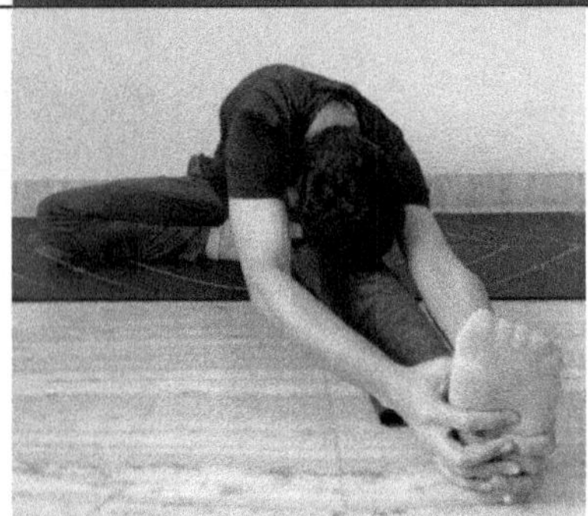
65. Shoulder stretch = kandharasana	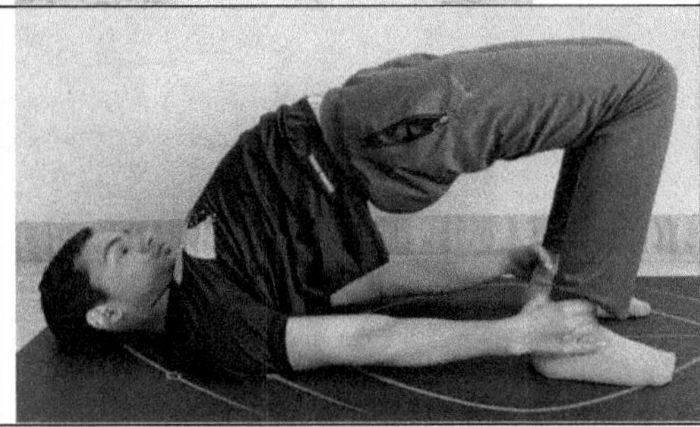

66. Cradling the baby

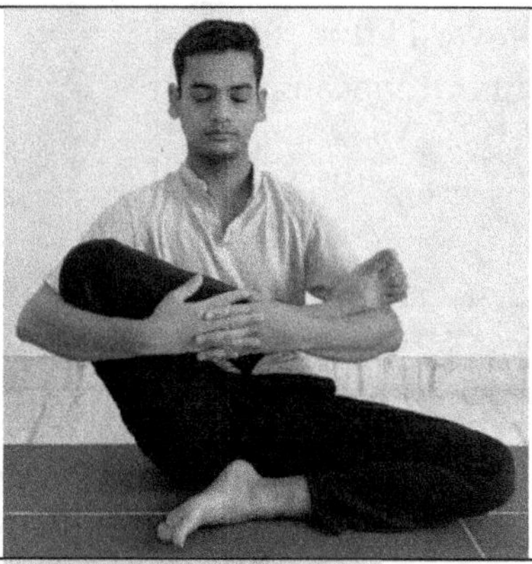

67. Pushing the wall

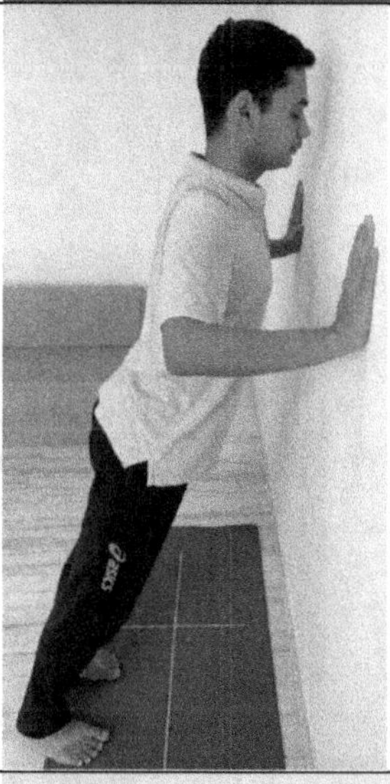

68. Butterfly = titliasana

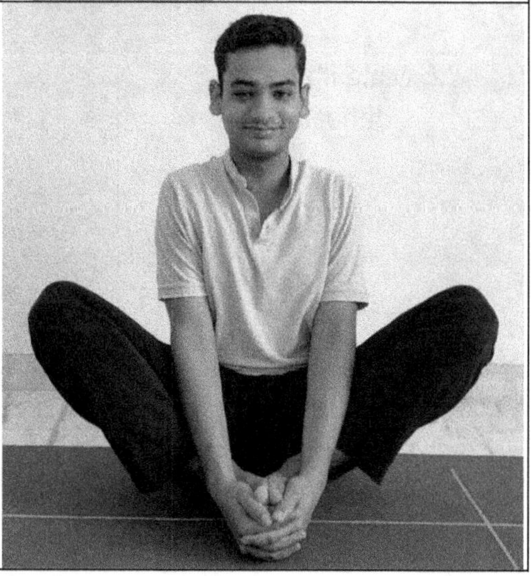

69. Upward lift = purvottanasana	
70. Back stretch = paschimottanasana	
71. Cow's face = gomukhasana	
72. Male libido = siddhasana	

73. Rooster = kukkutasana

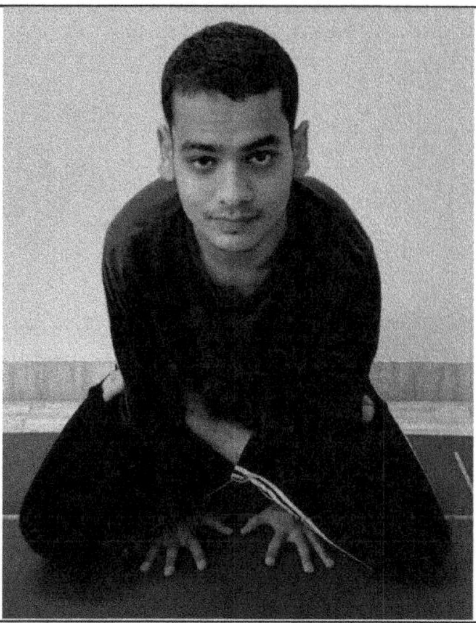

74. Tortoise = kurmasana

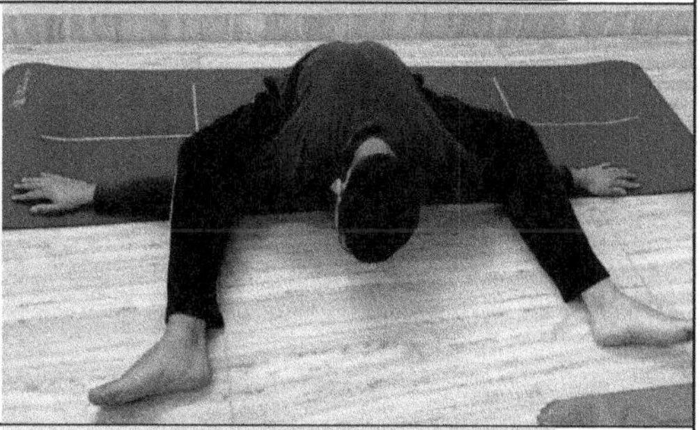

75. Raised Tortoise = uttana kurmasana

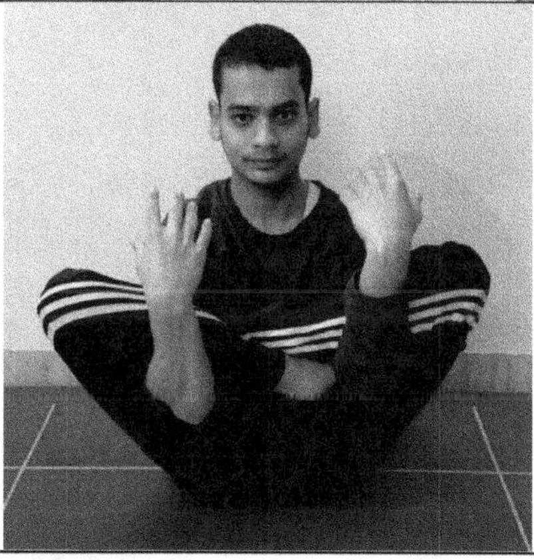

76. Frog = mandukasana	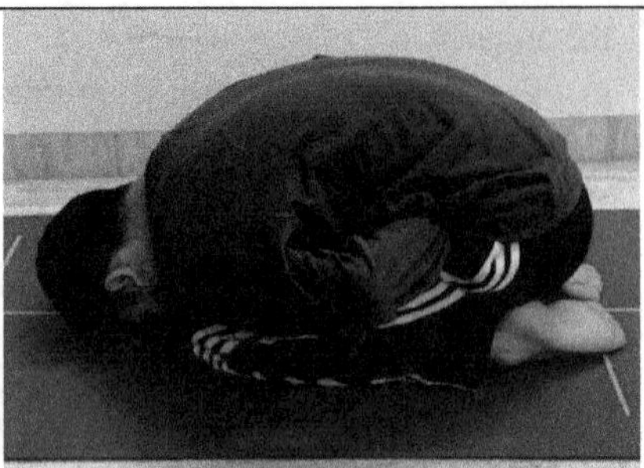
77. Raised Frog = uttana mandukasana	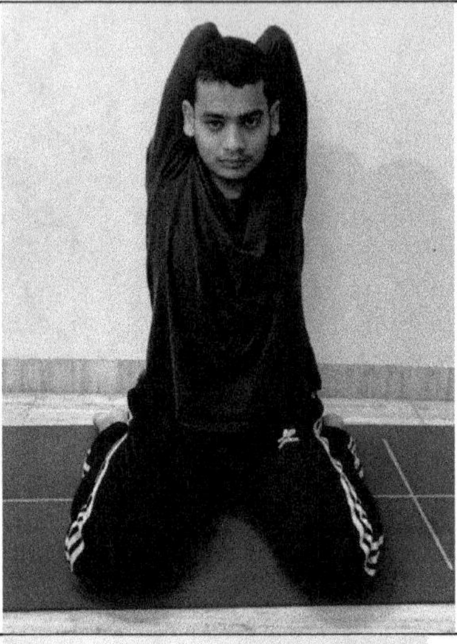
78. Sitting Brave = virasana	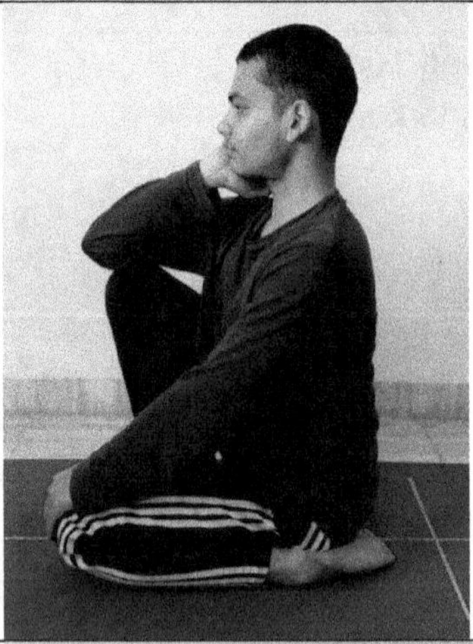
79. Sleeping thunderbolt = suptavajrasana	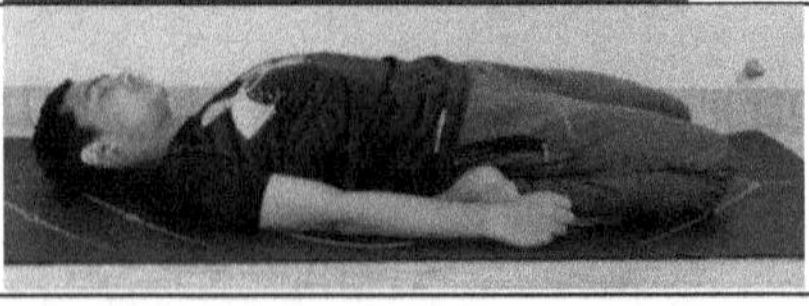

80. Peacock = mayurasana

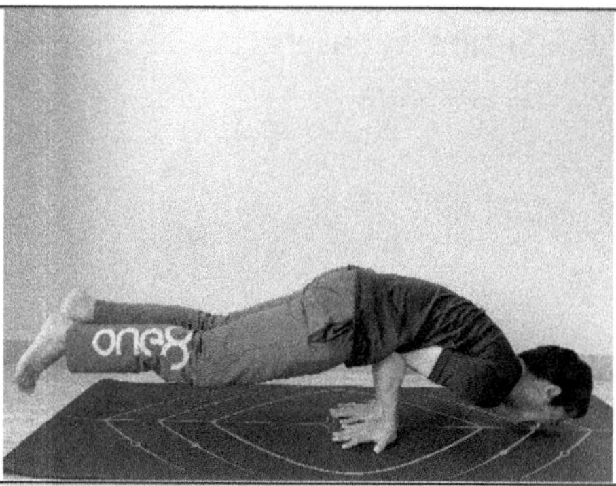

81. Crane = bakasana

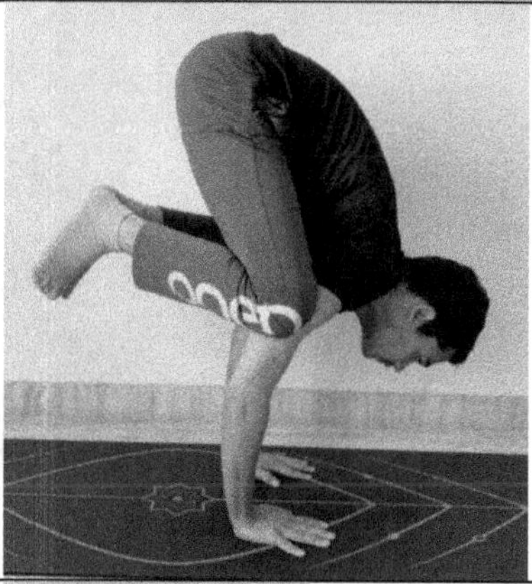

82. Headstand = sirshasana

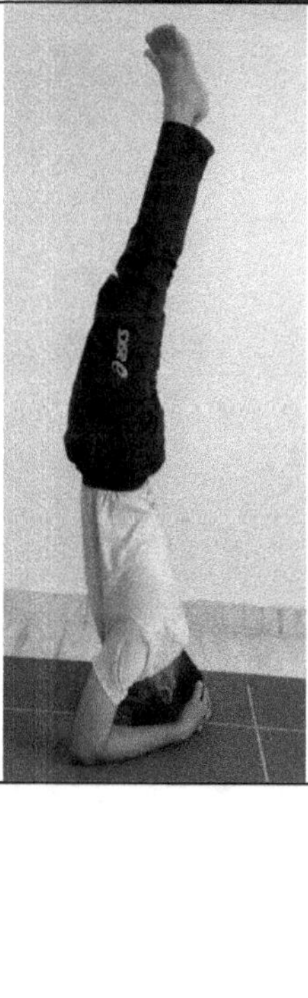

| 83. Sitting at ease = sukhasana | 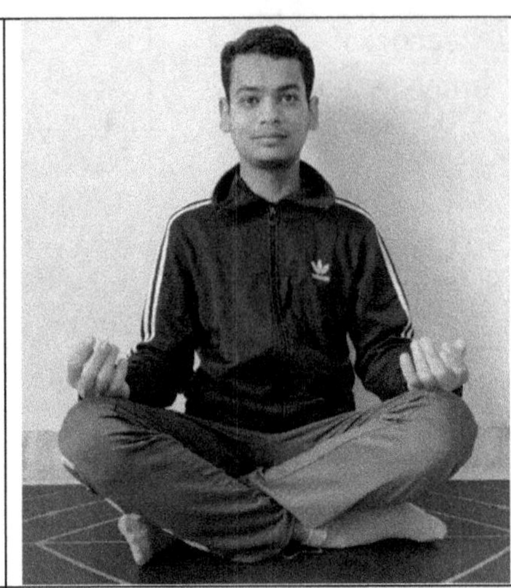 |
| 84. Thunderbolt = vajrasana | 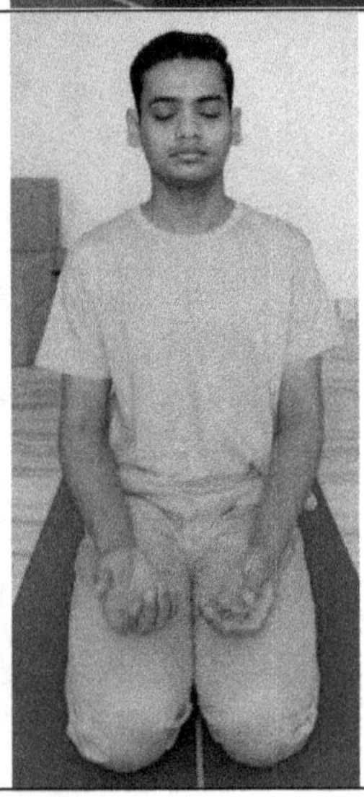 |

The 32 Asanas of Gheranda Samhita

Postures from Gheranda Samhita listed in the order of their description in the text (and not to mean the sequence of practice). The IAST transliteration is given along with the Sanskrit name.

Pose Name and literal Meaning	Pose	Remark
1. Siddhāsana सिद्धासन Perfect Pose		Left toe jutting out, Right toe inside calf. For men only. See 32 for females.
2. Padmāsana पद्मासन Lotus Pose		Both feet on opposite thighs
3. Bhadrāsana भद्रासन Strength Pose		Sitting on haunches with legs wide angled

4. Muktāsana मुक्तासन Freedom Pose		Both feet free. Right foot above thigh, left foot below thigh
5. Vajrāsana वज्रासन Thunderbolt Pose		Sitting on haunches with legs touching
6. Svastik-āsana स्वस्तिकासन Auspicious Pose		Both toes inside the bent knees
7. Siṃhāsana सिंहासन Lion Pose		Eyes wide, tongue stretched out

8. Gomukh-āsana गोमुखासन Cow's face Pose		One leg over the other, hands clasped behind back
9. Vīrāsana वीरासन Brave Pose		One knee up, the other leg folded on the ground under buttocks
10. Dhanur-āsana धनुरासन Bow Pose		Catch hold of the ankles and lift up on the navel
11. Śavāsana शवासन Corpse Pose		Lie down with arms and legs spread apart

12. Guptāsana गुप्तासन Hidden Pose		Hide both the feet inside the bent knees
13. Matsyāsana मत्स्यासन Fish Pose		Chest raised, neck bent, head touching the floor
14. (Ardha) Mats-yendrāsana (अर्ध) मत्स्येन्द्रासन Lord of the fish Pose		One knee up, the other on the floor, twist back
15. Paścim-ottānāsana पश्चिमोत्तानासन Back Stretch Pose		Reach forward to hold the feet, and touch the head to the knees

16. Gorakṣ-āsana गोरक्षासन Cowherd Pose	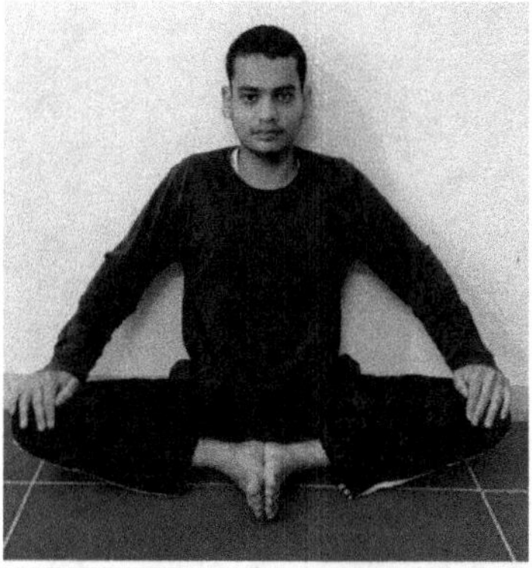	Soles touching, feet close to body
17. Utkaṭāsana उत्कटासन Chair Pose	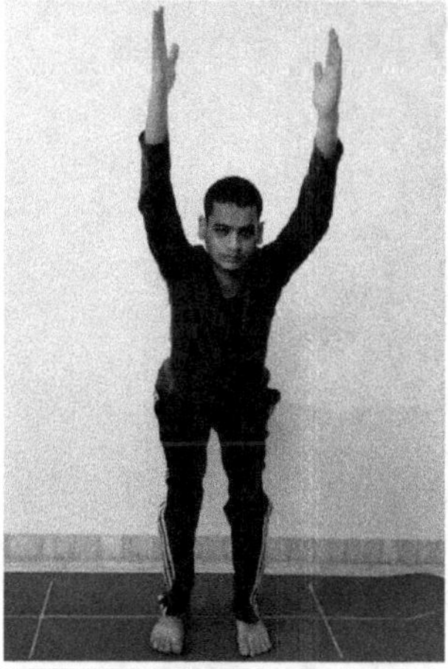	Stand with arms going up and knees slightly bent
18. Saṅkaṭāsana सङ्कटासन Danger Pose	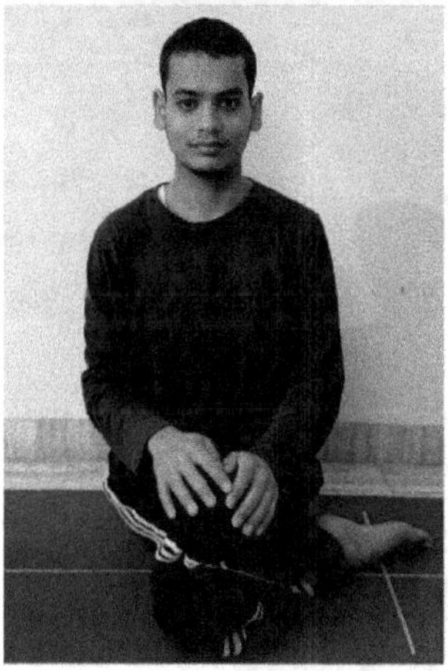	One knee folded above the other, as if accepting danger calmly

19. Mayūrāsana मयूरासन Peacock Pose	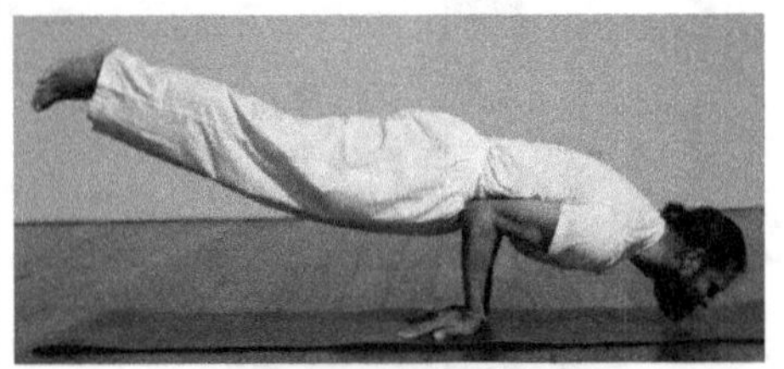	Hands towards feet, entire body up on palms
20. Kukkuṭāsana कुक्कुटासन Rooster Pose	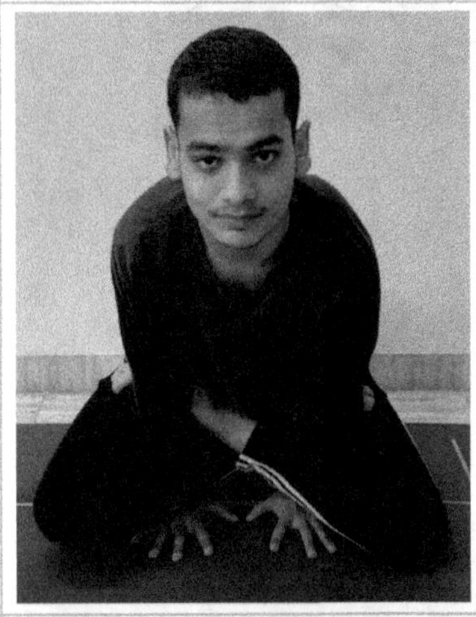	Lift body up on palms in padma-asana
21. Kūrmāsana कूर्मासन Tortoise Pose	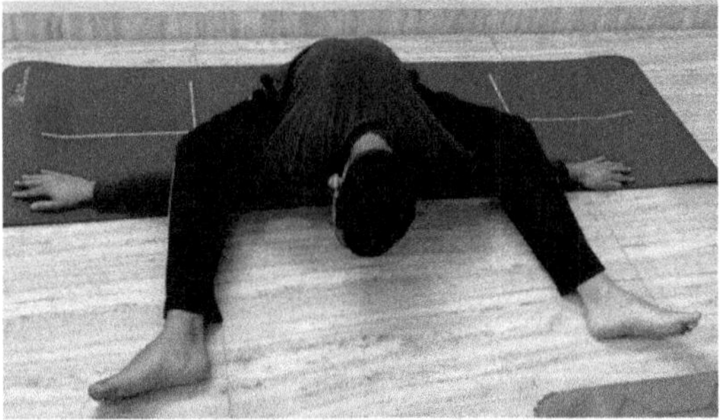	Sit with arms and legs spread-eagled
22. Uttāna kūrmāsana उत्तानकूर्मासन Raised Tortoise	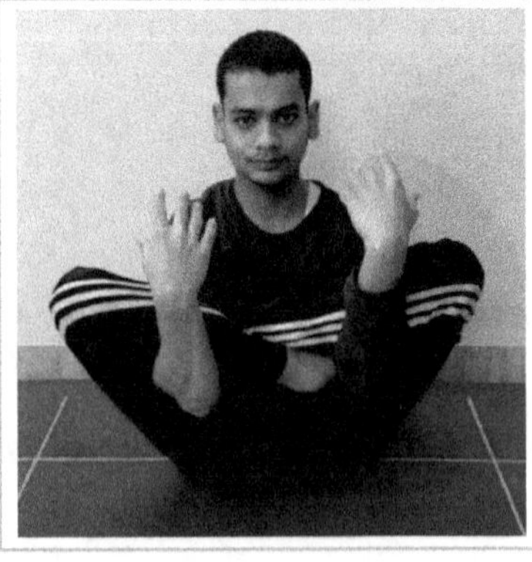	Sit in padma-asana with arms coming out from both calves

23. Maṇḍūk-āsana मण्डूकासन Frog Pose	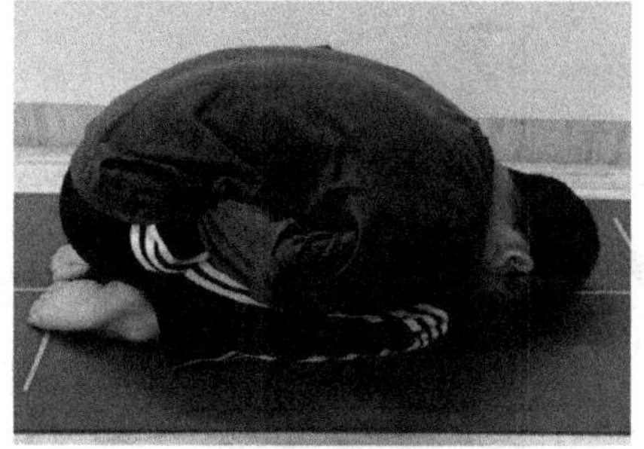	Bend in vajra-asana with hands in adi-mudra on thighs
24. Uttāna maṇḍūk-āsana उत्तान-मण्डूकासन Raised Frog	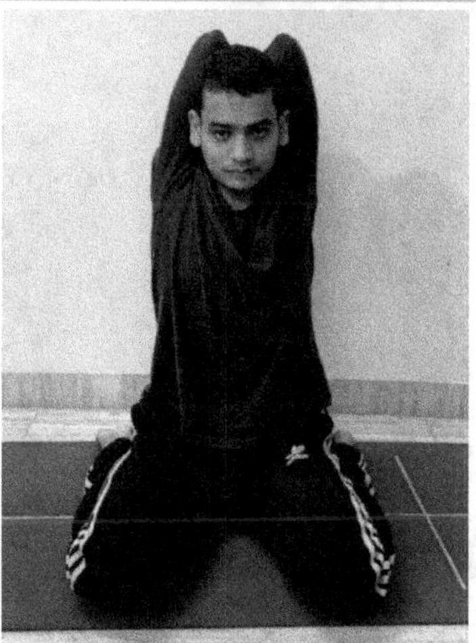	Feet besides the butttocks, arms raised up as in 3rd stage of pranayama
25. Vṛkṣāsana वृक्षासन Tree Pose	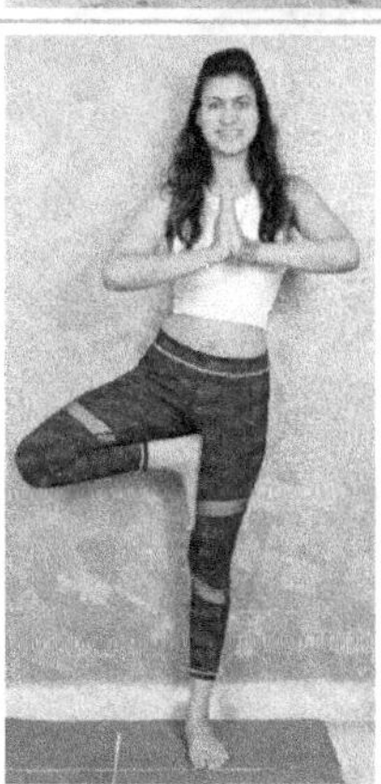	Stand with one leg joined to other thigh

26. Garuḍāsana गरुडासन Eagle Pose	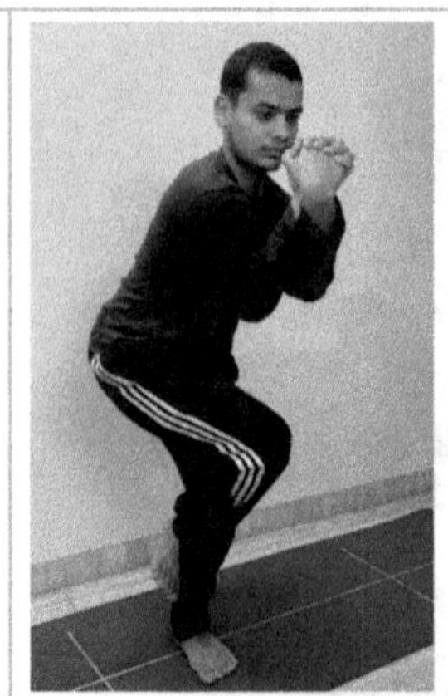	
27. Vṛṣabhāsana वृषभासन Bull Pose	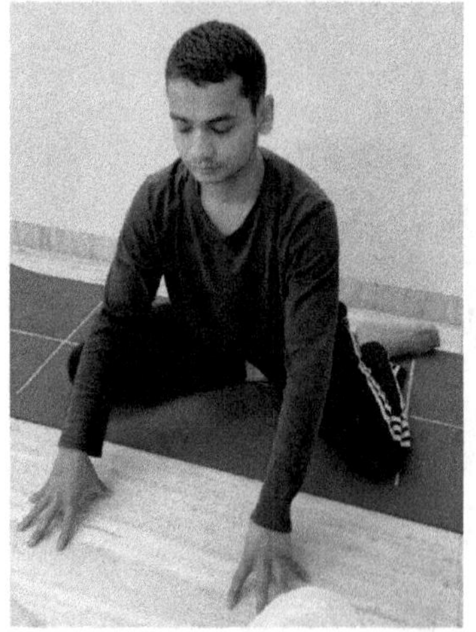	
28. Śalabhāsana शलभासन Locust Pose	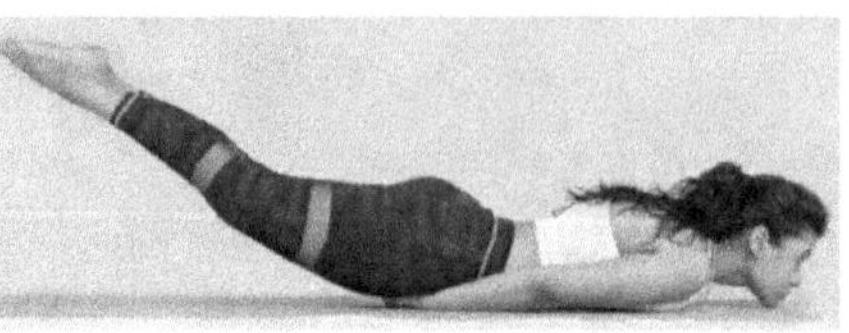	
29. Makarāsana मकरासन Crocodile Pose	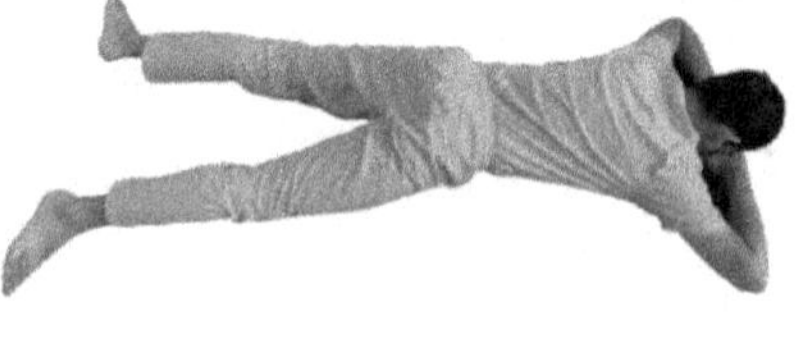	

30. Uṣṭrāsana उष्ट्रासन Camel Pose	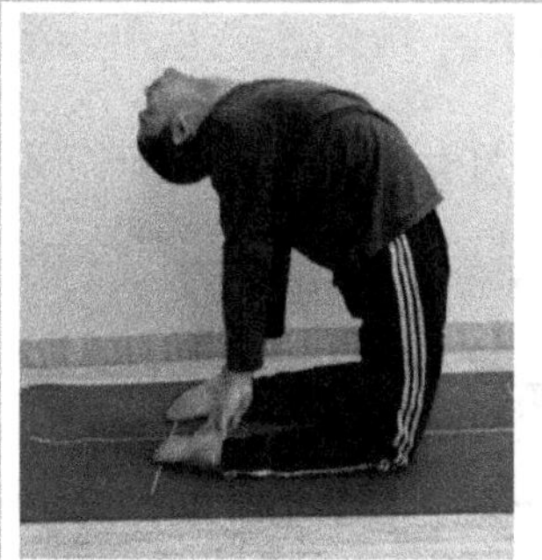	
31. Bhujaṅg- āsana भुजङ्गासन Cobra Pose	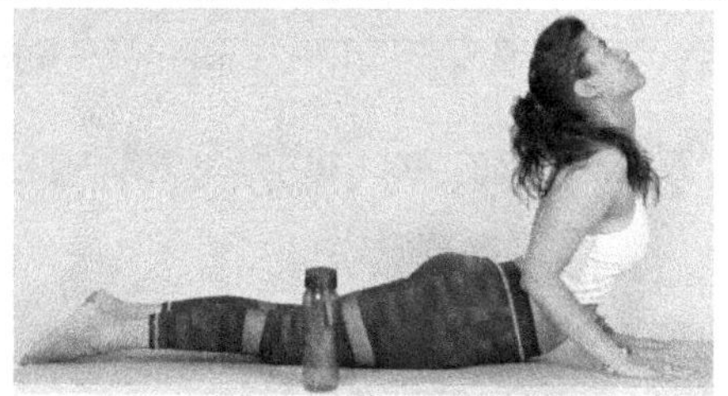	
32. Yogāsana योगासन Union Pose	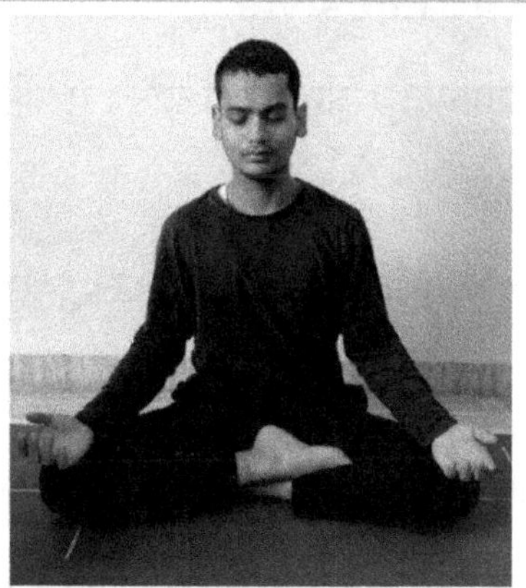	For both sexes. Similar to siddha-asana but we can reverse the legs, and toe does not jut out

Importance of Place, Time, Food, Seclusion

सुराज्ये धार्मिके देशे सुभिक्षे निरुपद्रवे । धनुः प्रमाण-पर्यन्तं शिलाग्नि-जल-वर्जिते ।
एकान्ते मठिका-मध्ये स्थातव्यं हठ-योगिना ॥ १२॥ HYP 1.12

आदौ स्थानं तथा कालं मिताऽहारं तथापरम् । नाडीशुद्धि ततः पश्चात्प्राणायामं च साधयेत्
॥ २॥ दूरदेशे तथाऽरण्ये राजधान्यां जनान्तिके । योगारम्भं न कुर्वीत कृतश्चेत्सिद्धिहा
भवेत् ॥ ३॥ अविश्वासं दूरदेशे अरण्ये रक्षिवर्जितम् । लोकारण्ये प्रकाशश्च तस्मात्त्रीणि
विवर्जयेत् ॥ ४॥ सुदेशे धार्मिके राज्ये सुभिक्षे निरुपद्रवे । तत्रैकं कुटिरं कृत्वा प्राचीरैः
परिवेष्टितम् ॥ ५॥ Gheranda Samhita 5.2

Importance of Specific Lifestyle

अत्याहारः प्रयासश्च प्रजल्पो नियमाग्रहः । जन-सङ्गश्च लौल्यं च षड्भिर्योगो विनश्यति ॥
१५॥ HYP 1.15

योगारम्भे वर्जयेच्च पथस्त्रीवह्निसेवनम् ॥ २६॥ Gheranda Samhita 5.26

तपः सन्तोष आस्तिक्यं दानमीश्वर-पूजनम् । सिद्धान्त-वाक्य-श्रवणं ह्रीमती च तपो हुतम्
। नियमा दश सम्प्रोक्ता योग-शास्त्र-विशारदैः ॥ १८॥ HYP 1.18

समाधिश्च परो योगो बहुभाग्येन लभ्यते । गुरोः कृपाप्रसादेन प्राप्यते गुरुभक्तितः ॥ १॥
विद्याप्रतीतिः स्वगुरुप्रतीतिरात्मप्रतीतिर्मनसः प्रबोधः । दिने दिने यस्य भवेत्स योगी
सुशोभनाभ्यासमुपैति सद्यः ॥ २॥ Gheranda Samhita 7.1

Importance of Outdoor Sports & Physical Activity

हठस्य प्रथमाङ्गत्वादासनं पूर्वमुच्यते । कुर्यात्तदासनं स्थैर्यमारोग्यं चाङ्ग-लाघवम् ॥ १९॥
HYP 1.19

आमं कुम्भमिवाम्भस्थो जीर्यमाणः सदा घटः ।
योगानलेन सन्दह्य घटशुद्धिं समाचरेत् ॥ ८॥ Gheranda Samhita 1.8

Gheranda Samhita Topic Matrix

The Gheranda Samhita is a manual of Hatha Yoga consisting of **351 stanzas** divided into **seven chapters** and enumerates **8 Topics**.

Chapter	Topic	Verses	Remarks
1	Introduction	1-11	Shatkarma = **Six Types of Cleaning** and scrubbing the body with water, air, thread, and cloth. Shatkarma is further sub-classified as Internal or External scrubbing.
	Shatkarma	12-60	
	I Dhauti	13	
	II Basti	45-49	
	III Neti	50-51	
	IV Lauliki	52	
	V Trataka	53-54	
	VI Kapalbhati	55-60	
2	**Asana**	1-45	32 **Body Postures**
3	**Mudra** & Bandha,	1-100	**Hand Gestures** & Muscle Locks, Mind **Imagination**
	Dharana	68-81	
4	**Pratyahara**	1-5	Turning **Senses Inwards**
5	**Pranayama**	1-96	**Breath Regulation**, Restraint and Control
	Seasons	10-15	
	Diet	16-32	
	Vayus	60-65	
6	**Dhyana**	1-22	**Meditation** through Contemplation
7	**Samadhi**	1-23	**Dissolving** into Infinity
(60+45+100+5+96+22+23) = 351 verses in all			

SaptaSadhana or SaptAnga are actually 7 + 1 = 8

Even though the Ashtanga or 8 Limbs of Yoga is a term made famous by Patanjali Yoga Sutras, commonly Saptanga or 7 limbs are attributed to the Gheranda Samhita. When we look through the Gheranda Samhita closely, we find that it also mentions 8 distinct limbs, albeit in a way that some early commentators overlooked it, and made 7 as its tenets.

- Patanjali mentions i) Yama ii) Niyama iii) Asana iv) Pranayama v) Pratyahara vi) Dharana vii) Dhyana viii) Samadhi.
- Gheranda elaborates i) Shatkarma ii) Asana iii) Mudra iv) Dharana v) Pratyahara vi) Pranayama vii) Dhyana viii) Samadhi.

The Yama and Niyama are not stated explicitly in Gheranda, albeit the Pupil himself has been named as the one who follows Yama and Niyama by default.

Though Shatkarma and Mudra have not been enumerated by Patanjali, these are implicit in his definition of Asana and Pranayama.

Patanjali Yoga Sutras

योगश्चित्तवृत्तिनिरोधः ॥ १.२ ॥ yogaścittavṛttinirodhaḥ । 1.2

योगः चित्त–वृत्ति–निरोधः ।

Yogic Life entails a Calming of the Processes in the Mind

1 Shatkarma for Purification – शौचः Shauca

2 Asana for Strengthening – दृढता Drdhata

3 Mudra & Bandha, Dharana for Endurance-स्थिरताSthirata

4 Pratyahara for Patience – धैर्य Dhairya

5 Pranayama for Lightness – आवरण क्षय Avaran Kshaya

6 Dhyana for Divine Meditation – दिव्य दृष्टि Divya Drishti

7 Samadhi = Dissolving in Bliss – योगः Yoga = Freedom from Duality

We have an anatomical body for which the Shatkarma and Asanas and Pranayama apply.
We also have an aural body for which the Pranayama, Mudra & Bandha, and Pratyahara apply.
Finally, there is the causal body which is adequately addressed by Dharana, Dhyana, Samadhi.

Chapter 1 – Shatkarma – Six Types of Cleansing

Chapter	Topic	Verses	Remarks
1	Introduction	1-11	Shatkarma = Six
	Shatkarma	12-44	types of cleaning
	I Dhauti	13	and scrubbing
	Agnisara	20	the body with
	Stomach/Colon	23-24	water, air,
	Teeth/Gums	26-28	thread, and
	Tongue	29	cloth.
	Ears	33	
	Food Pipe	36-37	
	Colon		
	II Basti	45-49	Throat
	III Neti	50-51	Nose
	IV Lauliki	52	Diaphragm
	V Trataka	53-54	Eyes
	VI Kapalbhati	55-59	Forehead

I Dhauti - 13 Types – Teeth etc. Cleansing

II Basti - 12 Types – Throat/Lungs/Stomach Cleansing

III Neti - 1 Type – Nostrils Cleansing

IV Lauliki (Nauli) - 1 Type – Diaphragm Cleansing

V Trataka - 1 Type – Eyes (Thoughts) Cleansing

VI Kapalbhati - 3 Types – Tissues Cleansing

Chapter 2 – Asana – Thirty Two Types of Body Postures

Verse	Topic – Asana Name	Asana No	English Name
2.1	the 84 lakh asanas or yonis	-	Anatomy Types
2.2	the 84 standard poses	-	84 Poses
2.3-6	the 32 Asanas named	-	32 Poses
2.7	Siddhasana	1	Perfect Pose
2.8	Padmasana	2	Lotus
2.9-10	Bhadrasana	3	Strength
2.11	Muktasana / Sukhasana	4	Freedom / Easy
2.12	Vajrasana	5	Thunderbolt
2.13	Swastikasana	6	Auspicious
2.14-15	Simhasana	7	Lion
2.16	Gomukhasana	8	Cow's Face
2.17	Virasana	9	Brave
2.18	Dhanurasana	10	Bow
2.19	Shavasana	11	Corpse
2.20	Guptasana	12	Hidden
2.21	Matsyasana	13	Fish
2.22-23	Matsyendrasana	14	Lord of Fish
2.24	Paschimottanasana	15	Back Stretch
2.25-26	Gorakshasana	16	Cowherd
2.27	Utkatasana	17	Chair
2.28	Sankatasana	18	Danger
2.29-30	Mayurasana	19	Peacock
2.31	Kukkutsana	20	Rooster
2.32	Kurmasana	21	Tortoise
2.33	Uttana Kurmasana	22	Raised Tortoise
2.34	Mandukasana	23	Frog
2.35	Uttana Mandukasana	24	Raised Frog
2.36	Vrikshasana	25	Tree
2.37	Garudasana	26	Eagle
2.38	Vrishabasana / Vrishasana	27	Bull
2.39	Shalabhasana	28	Locust
2.40	Makarasana	29	Crocodile
2.41	Ushtrasana	30	Camel
2.42-43	Bhujangasana	31	Cobra
2.44-45	Yogasana	32	Yogic

01 Siddhasana

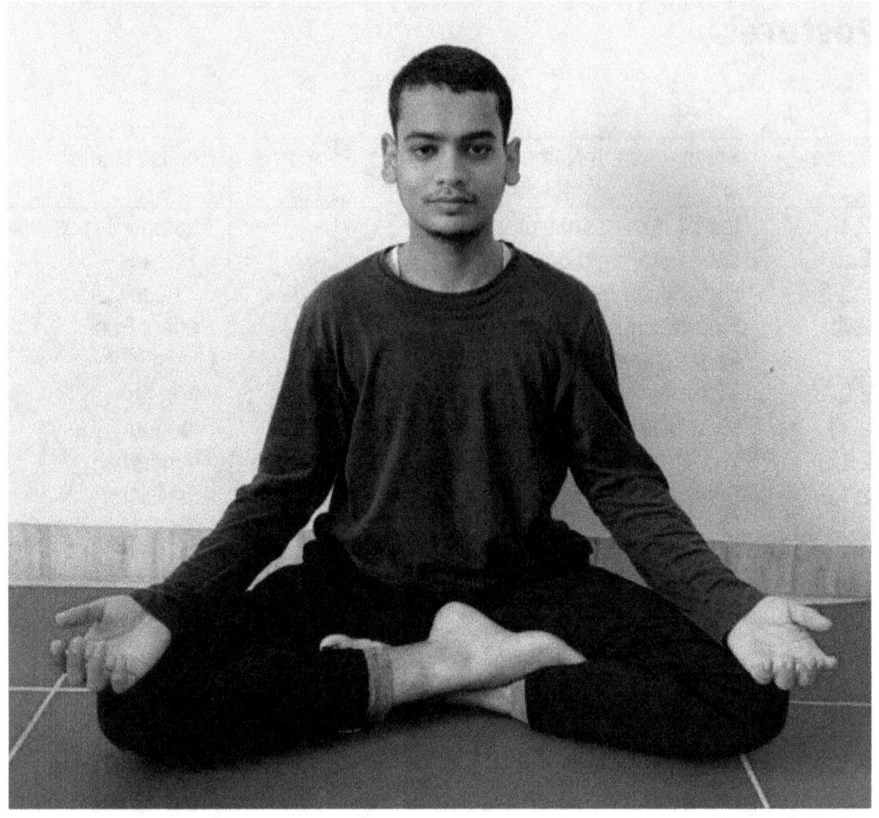

Recommended only for men as it activates masculine hormones.
Left leg is below. Do not do it with alternate leg position.
Left heel presses the male organ.
Right foot is placed directly above the left foot.
Left toe is protruding outside the right calf.
Right toe is hidden inside the left calf.

02 Padmasana

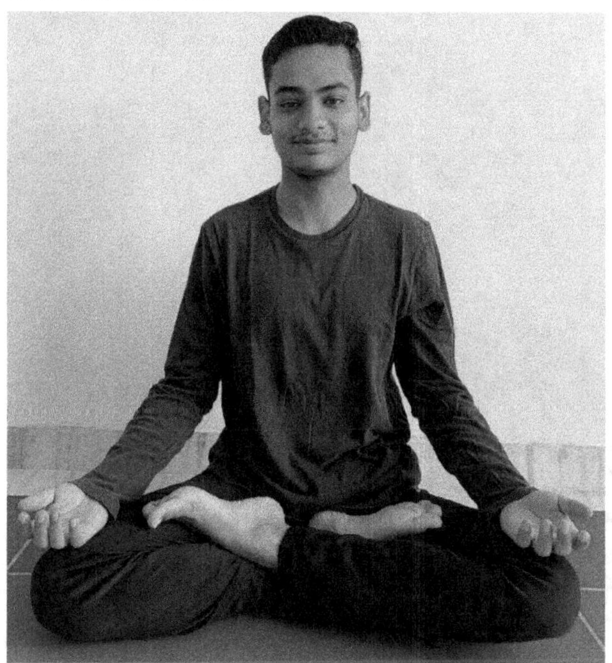

FEET rested comfortably on either THIGH.

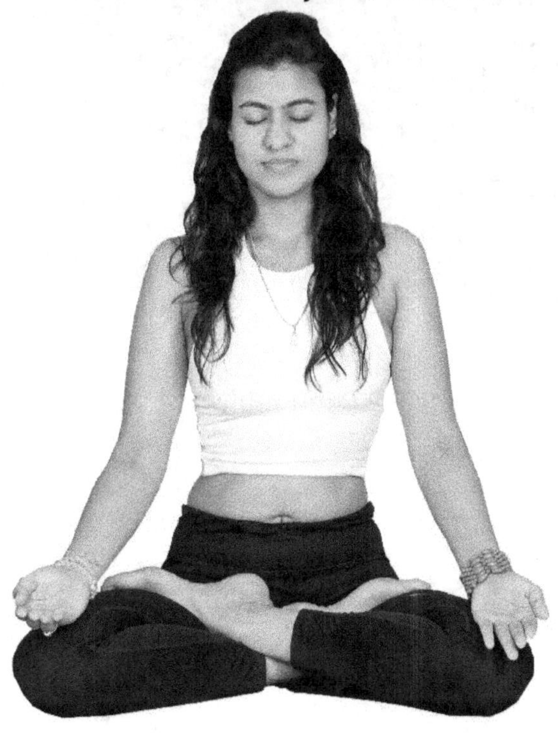

03 Bhadrasana

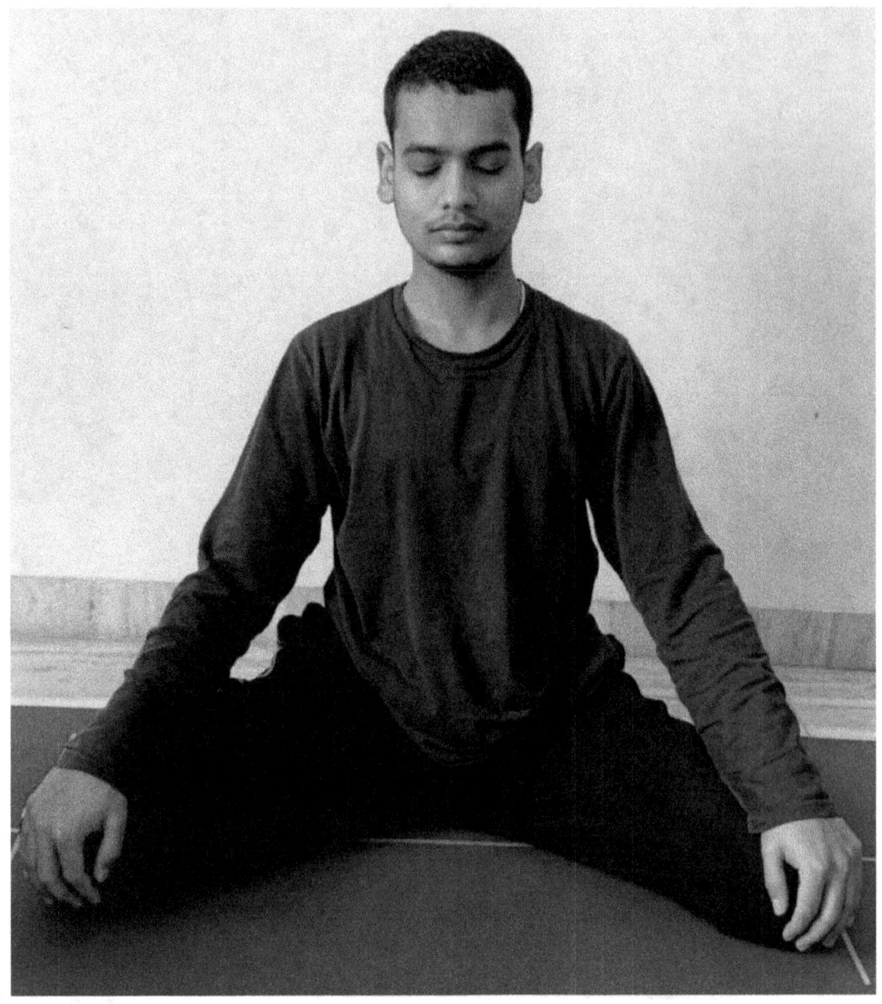

Feet are under buttocks.
Legs spread out in as wide an angle as comfortable.

04 Muktasana / Sukhasana

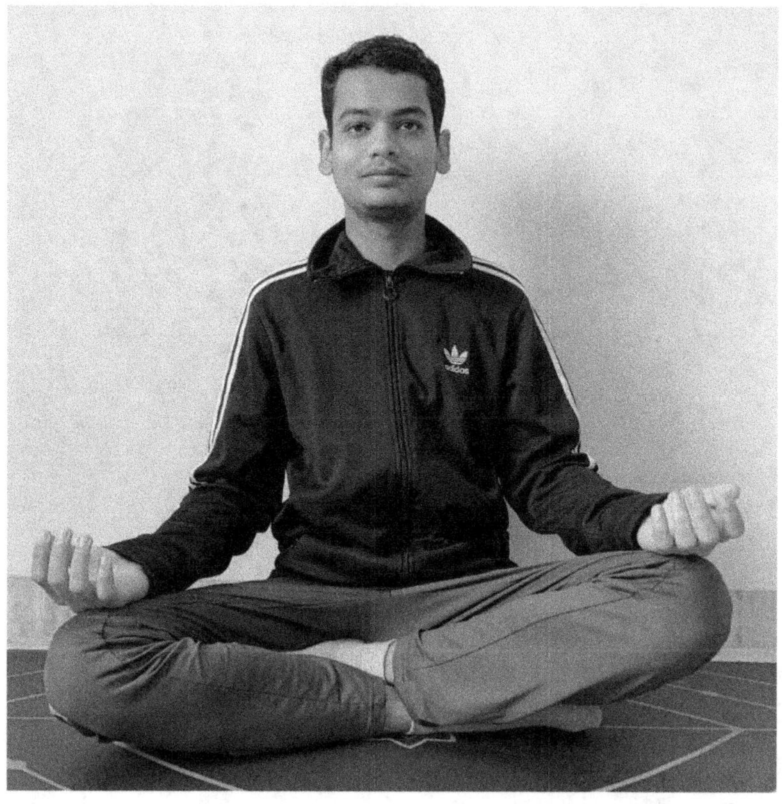

Simple cross-legged posture that we all enjoy sitting in. For most of us this is the standard sitting pose for our Pranayama and Meditation practices.

Can be done with either leg on top as comfortable.

05 Vajrasana

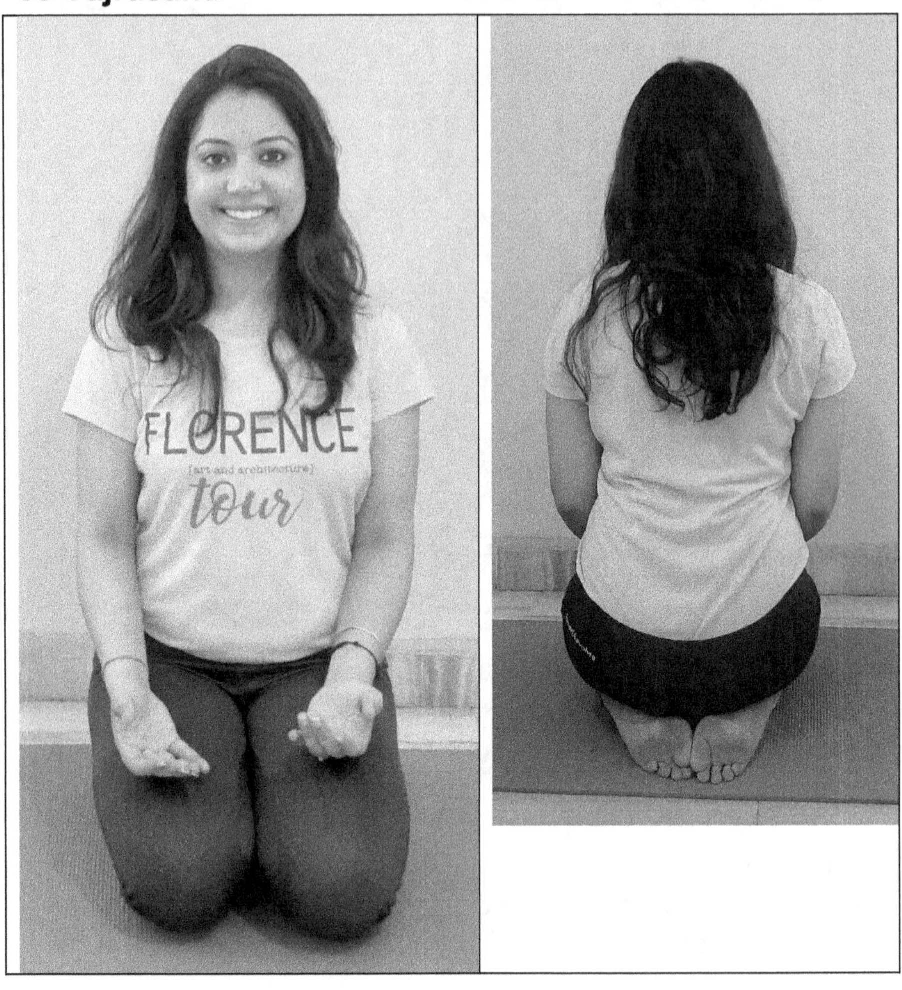

Feet under the buttocks. Recommended pose for Ujjayi or
Bhastrika Pranayama.

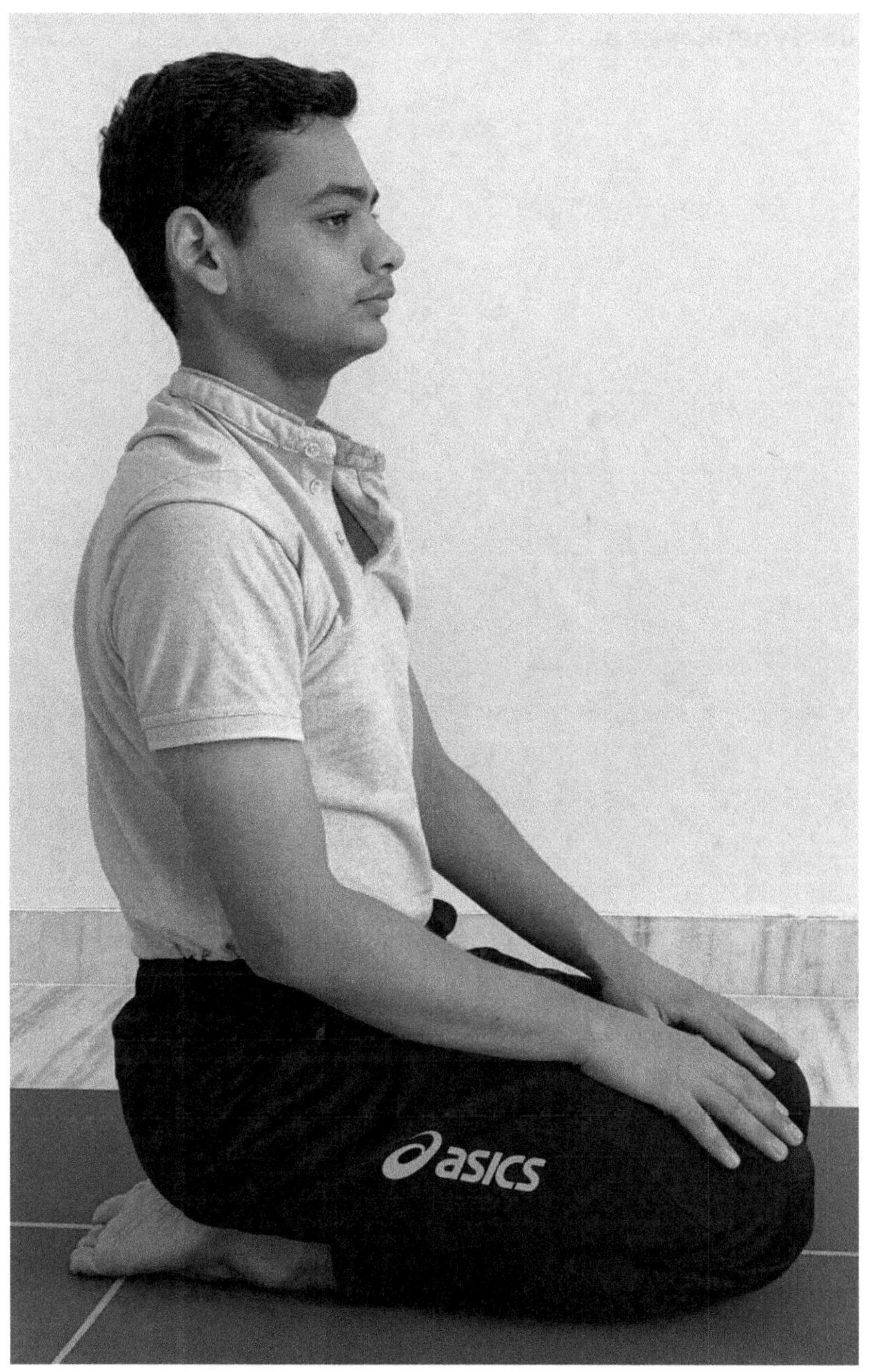

06 Svastikasana

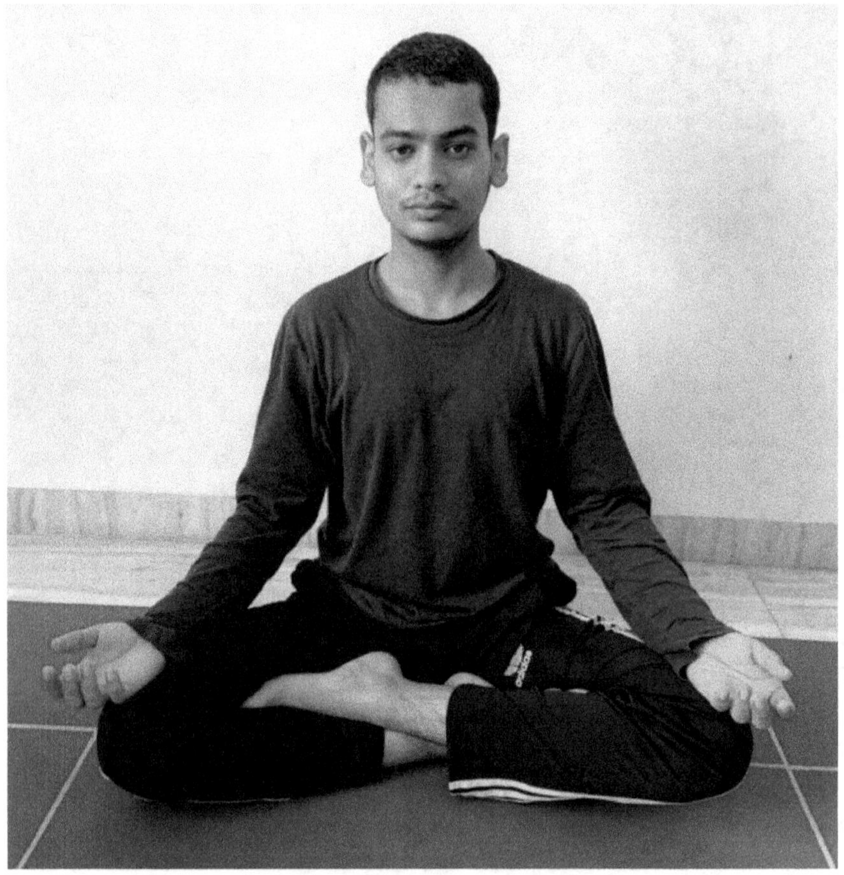

Feet position are different from other similar postures.

A cross-legged position where the feet are comfortably placed touching the thighs, rather than under the thighs as in Muktasana/Sukhasana.

Can be done with either leg on top as comfortable.

07 Simhasana

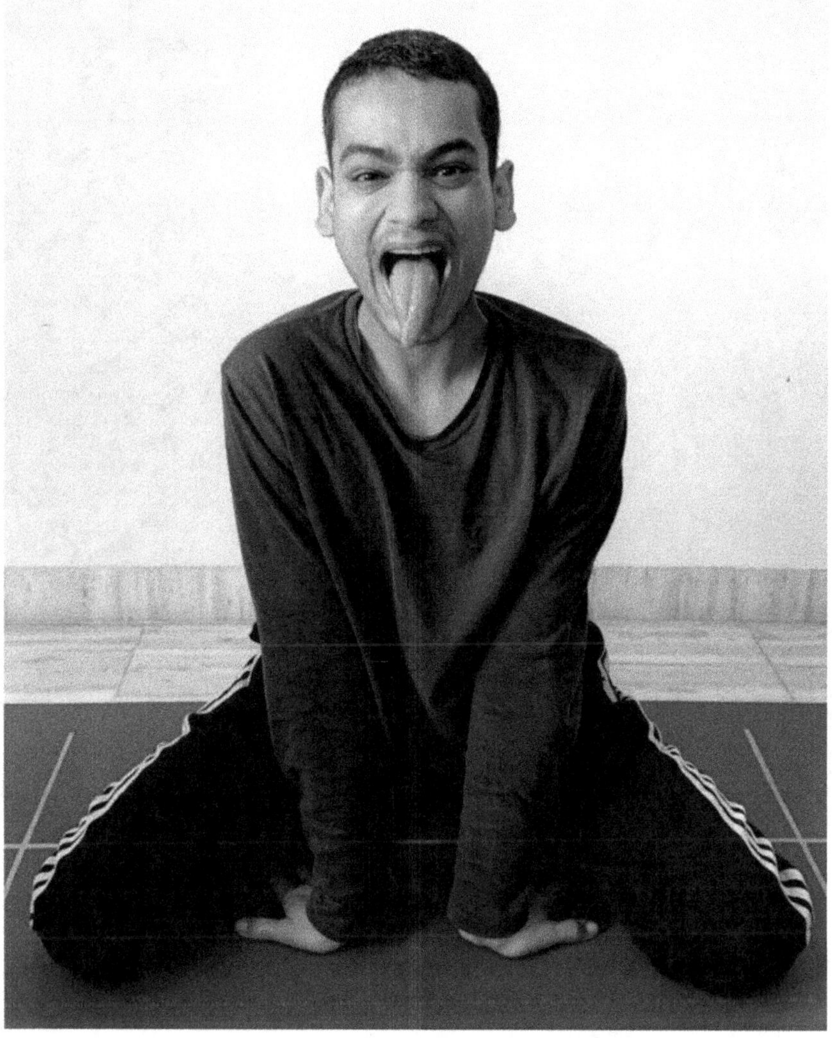

With lots of effort on the throat and face muscles, we stretch the tongue out and open the eyes wide, mimicking a roaring lion.

Sitting posture can be changed as it is comfortable to the student, the pose shown here is only a sample that helps exert maximum pressure.

08 Gomukhasana

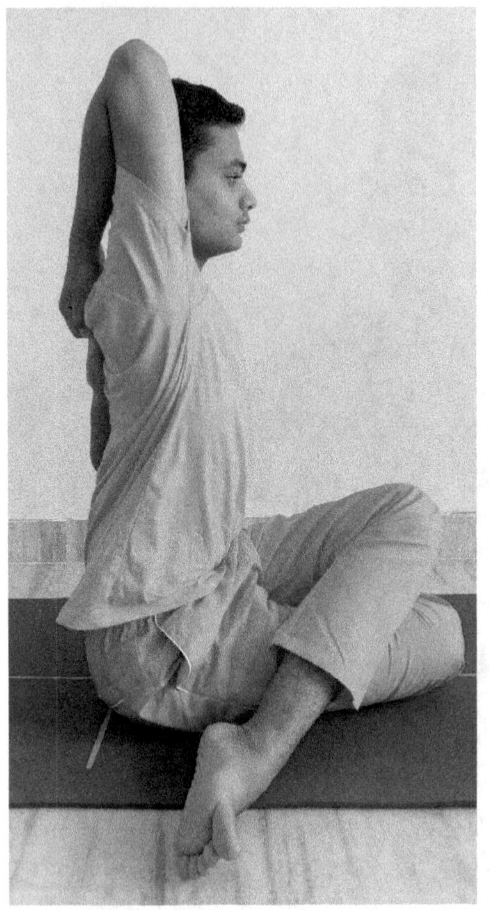

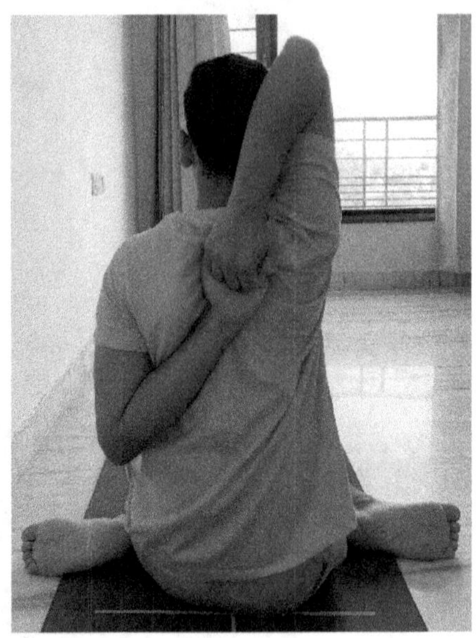

With folded legs placed one over the other, the hands are clasped
behind the back.

Can be done with either leg on top as comfortable.

09 Virasana

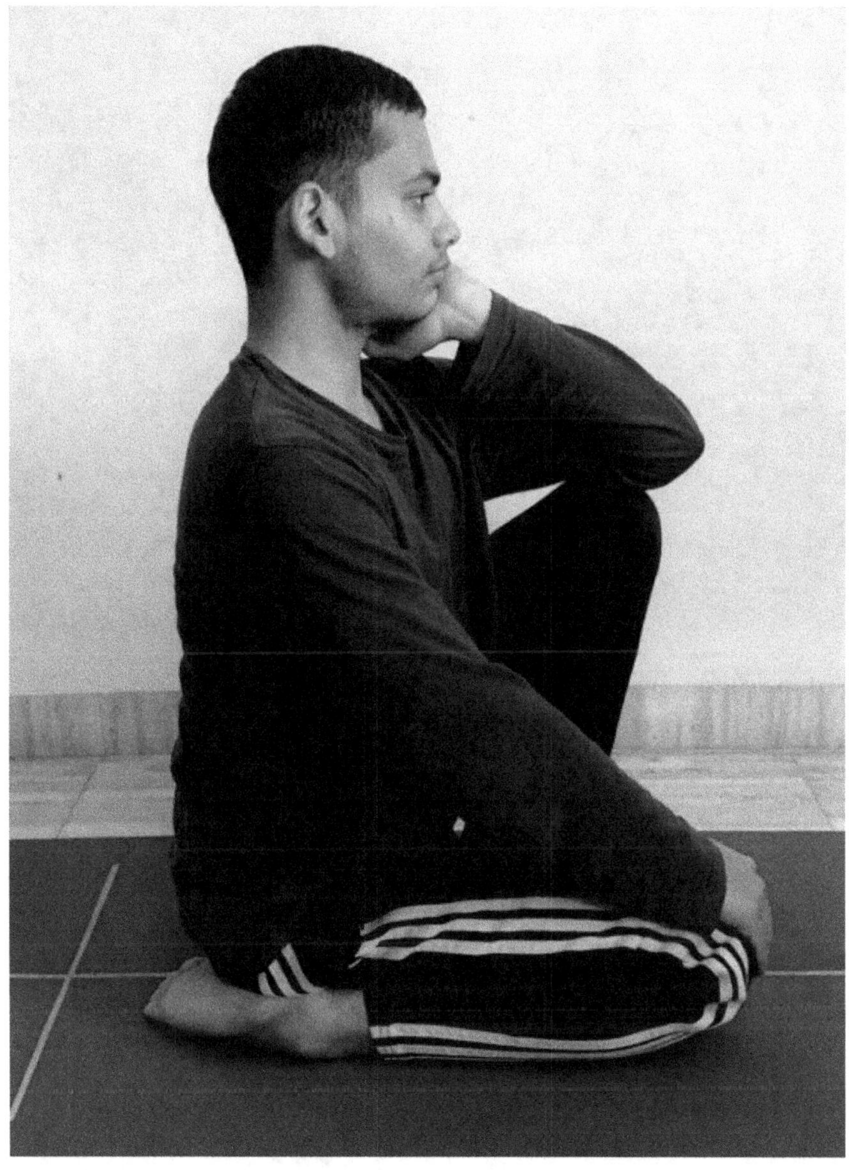

Sitting on right foot with right leg folded on ground. Left elbow resting on left knee. Right hand on right knee.

Can be done with either leg on top as comfortable.

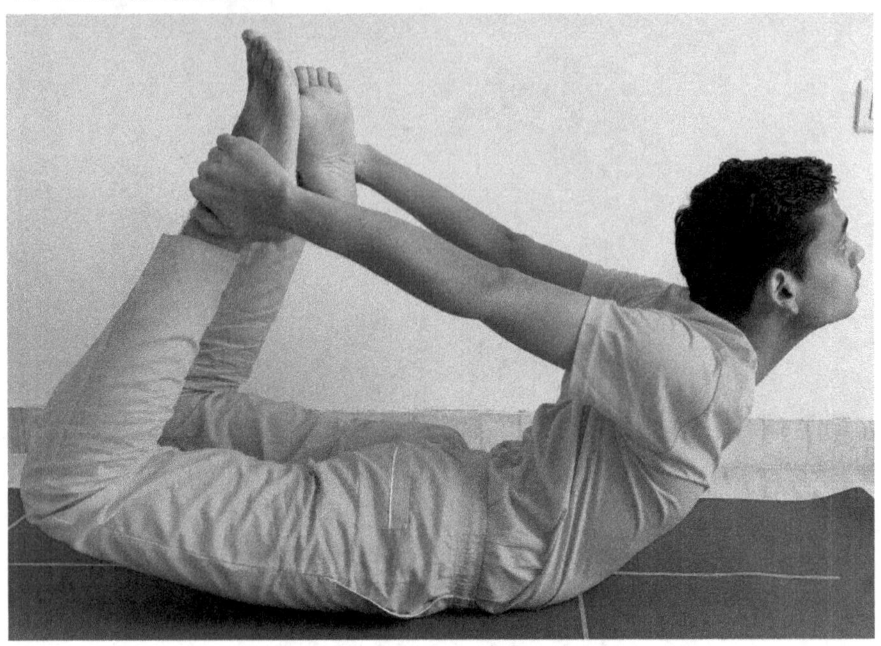

Hold the ankles and lift up on the navel. Look up.
Whole body is taut in a nice curve.

11 Shavasana

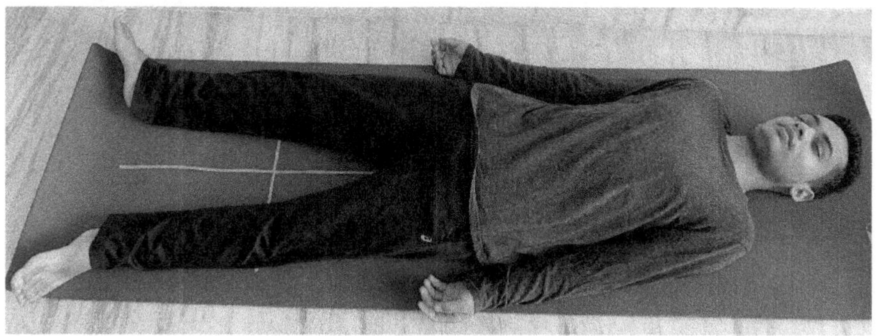

Rest comfortably on the floor. Arms are near the body with palms facing up. Feet are outstretched with toes pointing outwards. Entire body is loose yet still.

12 Guptasana

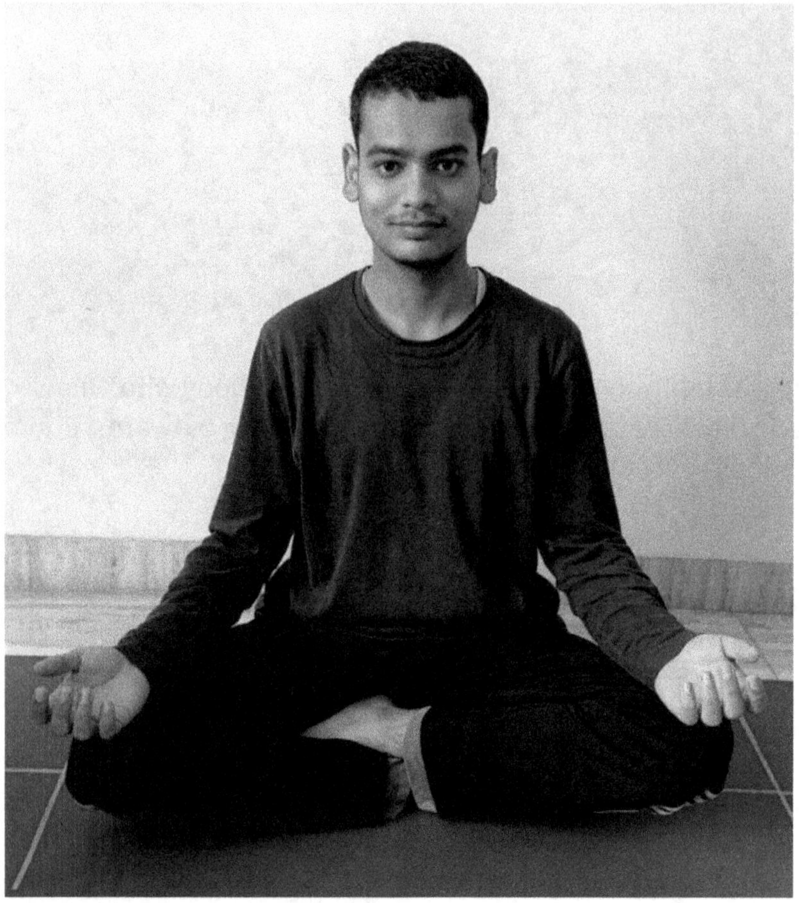

Feet are hidden inside both calves. Resembles Siddhasana, but can be done by both males and females.

Can be done with either leg on top as comfortable.

13 Matsyasana

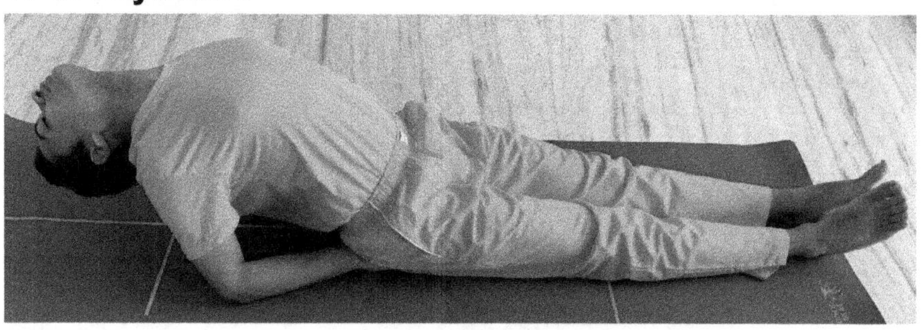

Chest lifted up fully, head resting on the floor with a steady neck.

14 Matsyendrasana

Ardha Matsyendrasana

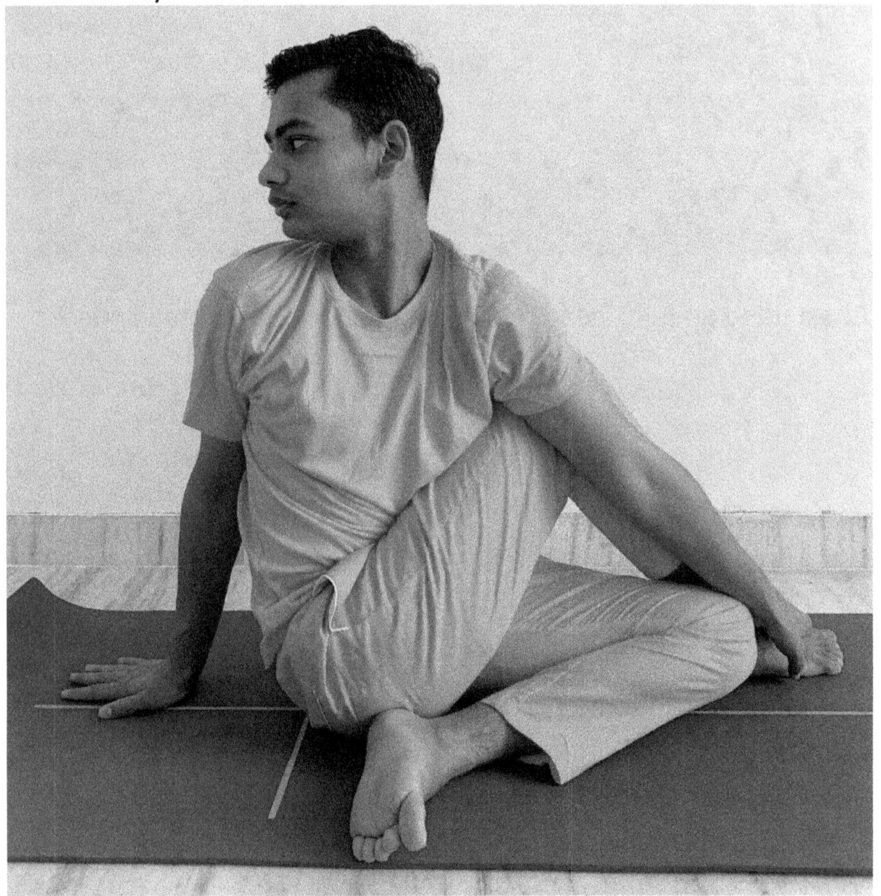

Thigh and knee of one leg presses firmly against the stomach and abdomen due to pressure lock of the arm, and the spine is nicely twisted.

Should be done with either leg on top, one after the other, so these are two asanas actually.

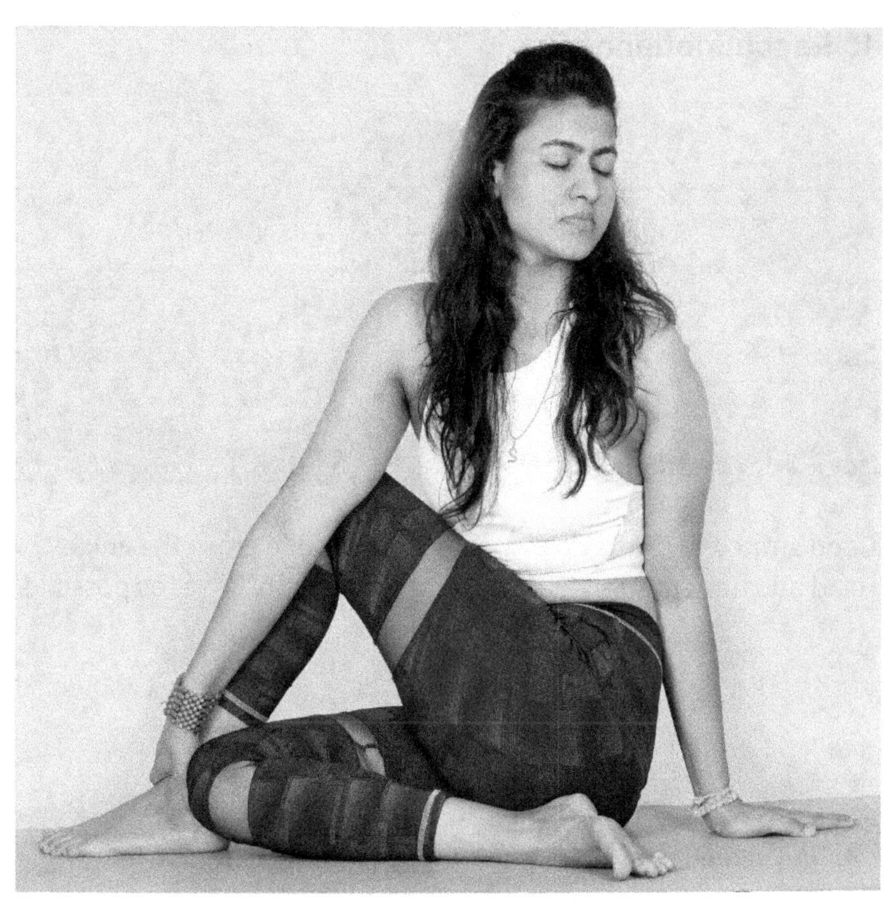

15 Paschimottanasana

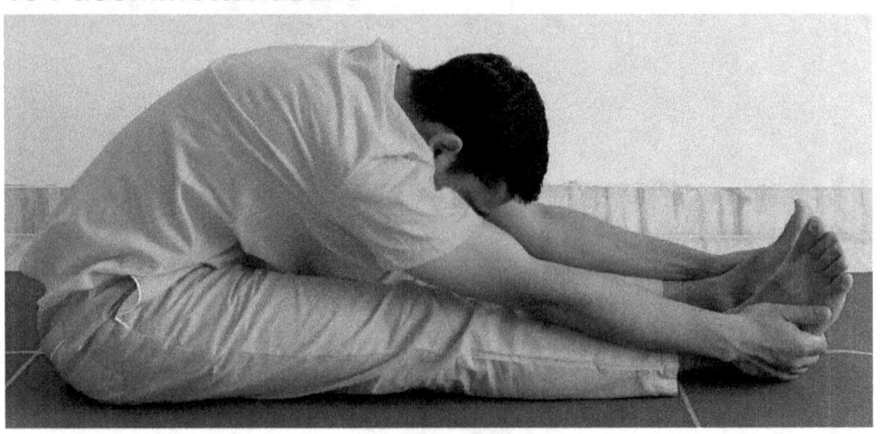

Good stretch to the back as we reach forward to grasp the ankles.
Head and neck in straight line and as close to the knees as possible.

16 Gorakshasana

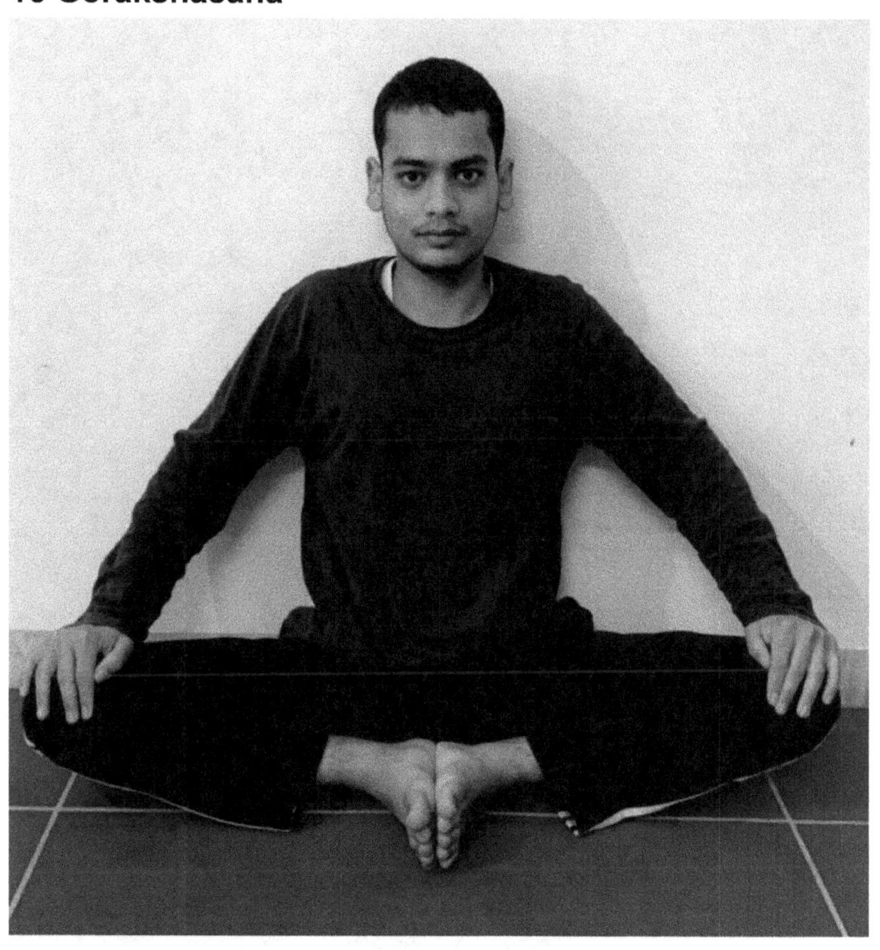

Soles of feet joined perfectly.
Legs as close to the body as comfortable.
Hands resting on knees.

17 Utkatasana

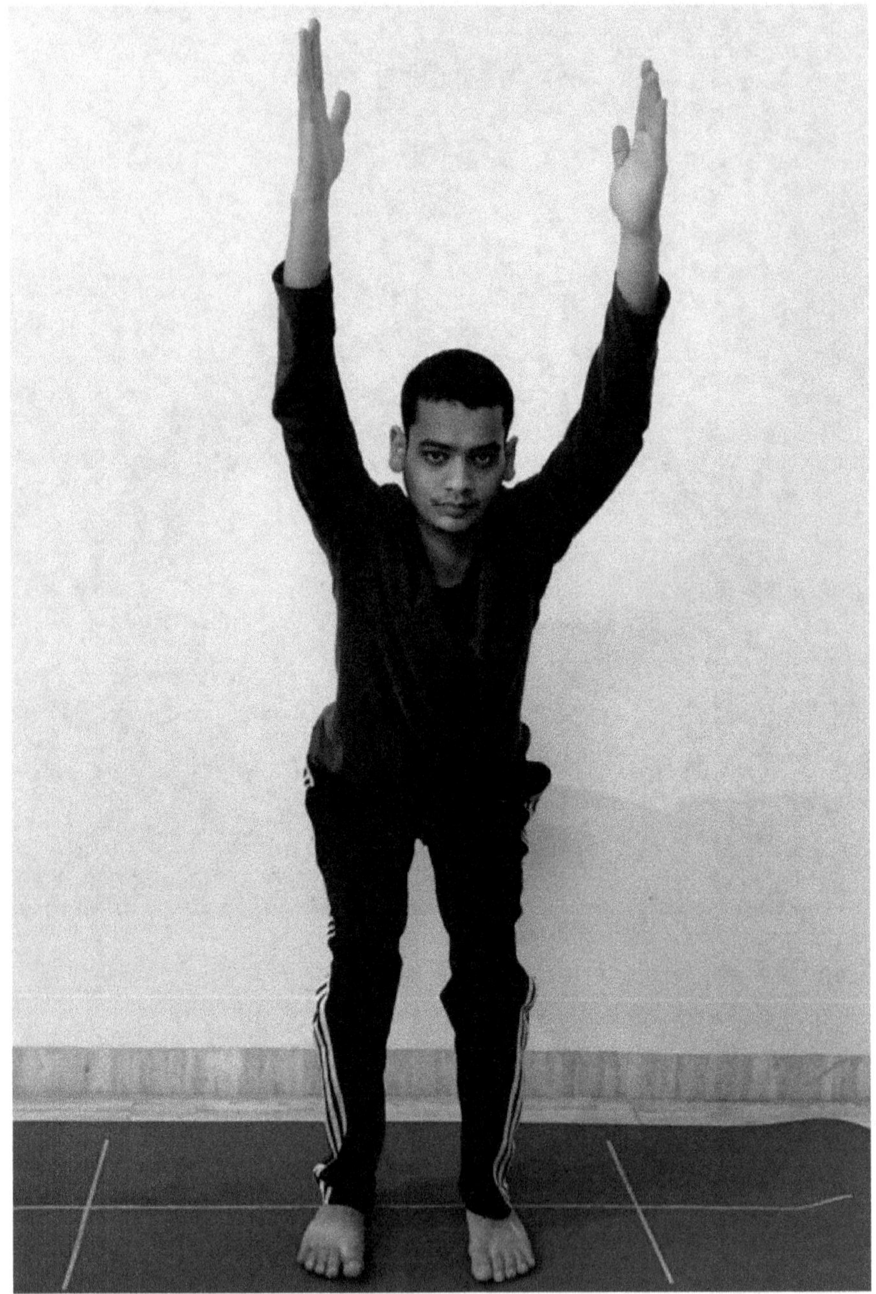

Sitting on an imaginary chair, with pressure on the knees, hands adjusted for stability.

18 Sankatasana

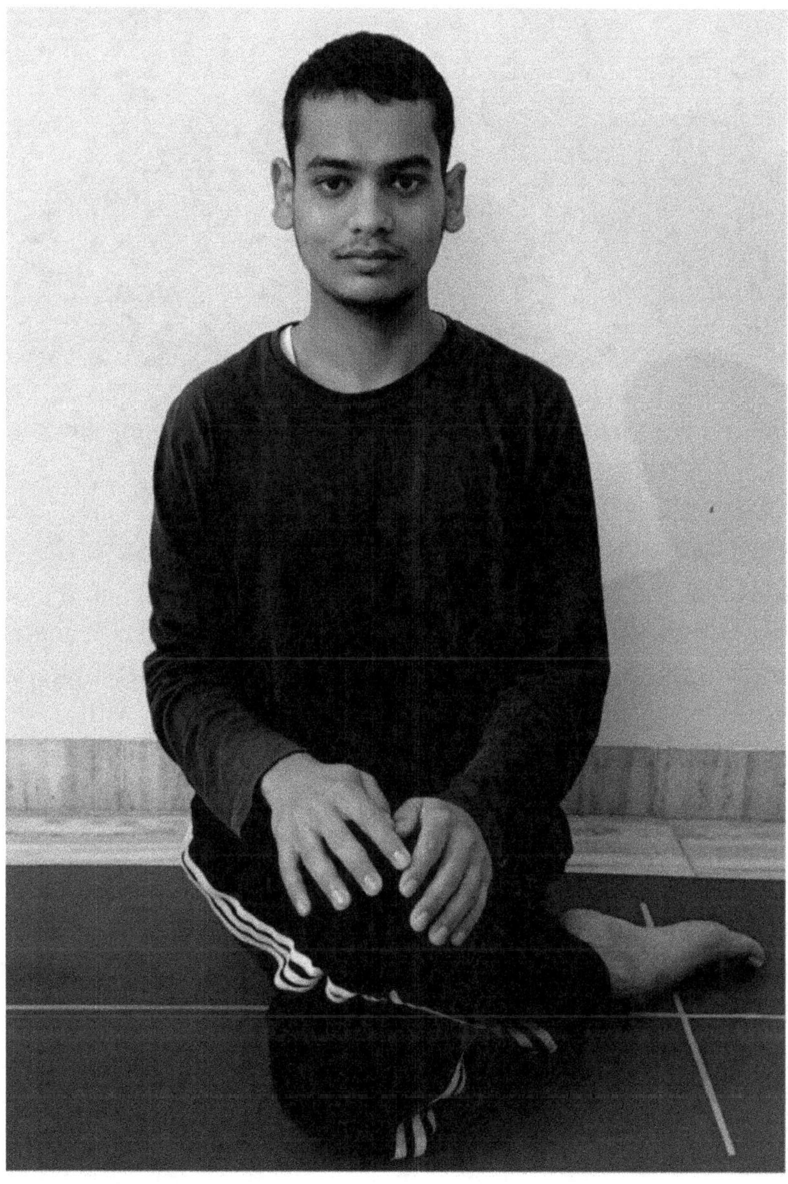

A posture to feel defensive amidst a crisis, legs folded on top of each other to represent the shrinking mind. Sit on one buttock. Can interchange the legs as per comfort.

19 Mayurasana

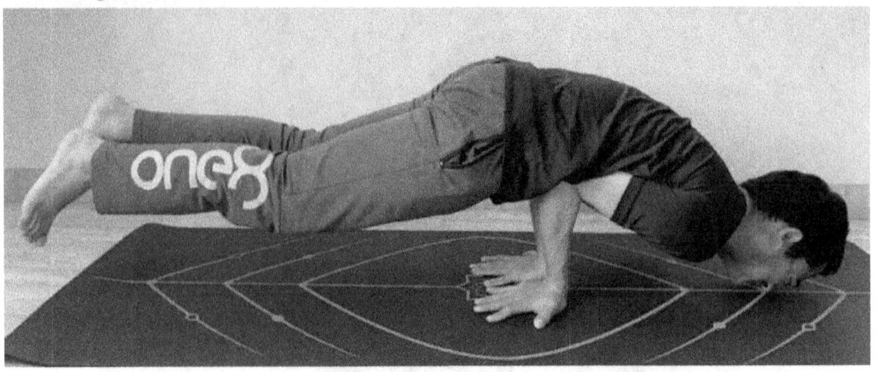

An advanced posture for those who are very fit or practicing since youth.

Kneel on the floor, keeping feet close to each other.
Make the knees apart and lunge forward.
Place the hands facing down and fingers pointing towards the feet.
Join both wrists and keep arms close to each other for better lift.
Now go forward and lift the whole body up on the palms, with elbows sticking into the abdomen.

20 Kukkutasana

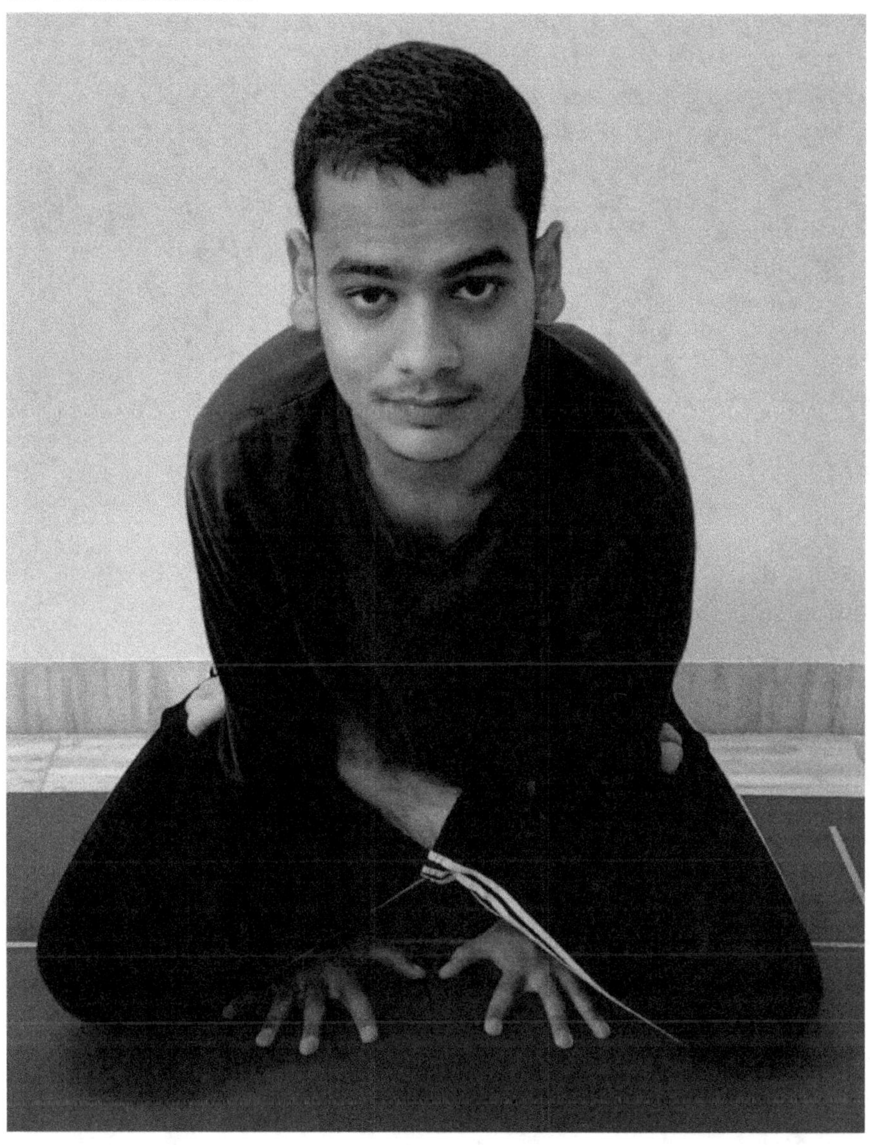

Sit in Padmasana with arms through the calves, palms outstretched on the floor. Lift the body up on both palms.

An advanced posture for those who are very fit or practicing since childhood.

21 Kurmasana

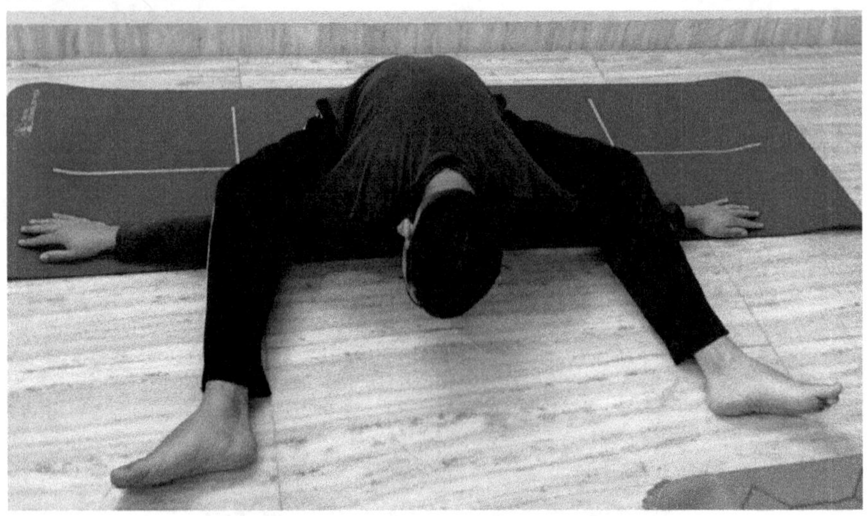

Legs outstretched in front, arms stretched out under the legs on either side. Go forward to touch the floor if possible.

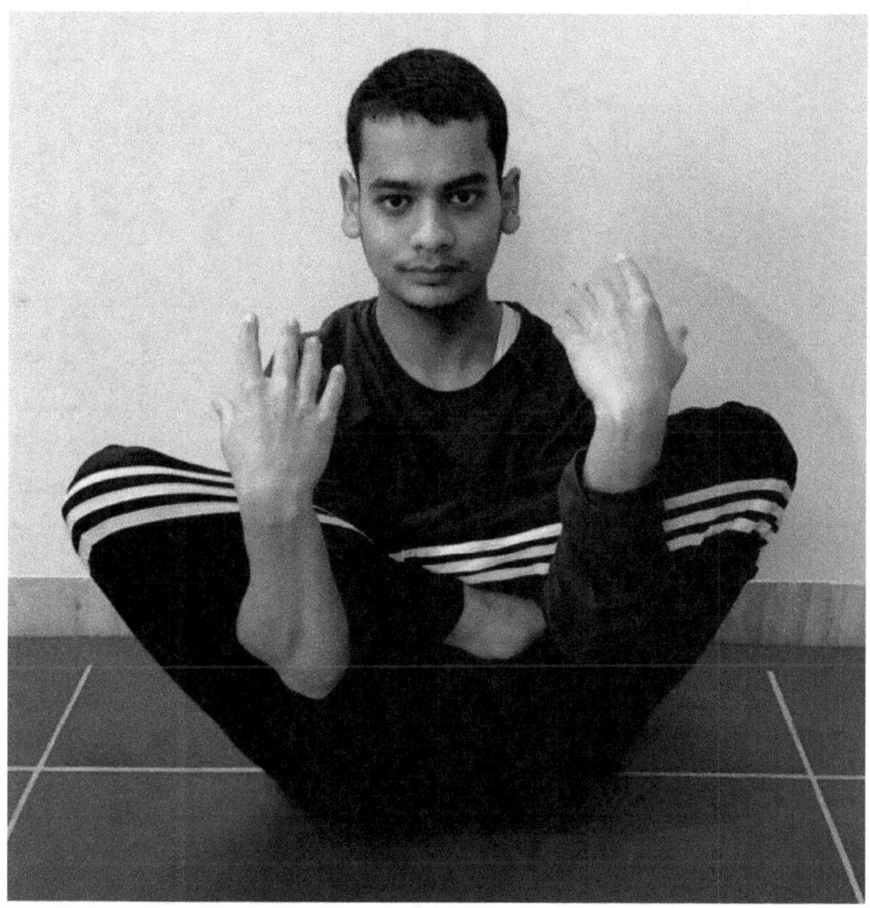

An advanced posture for those who are very fit or practicing since youth.

Resembles the Kukkutasana, wherein the palms are on the floor, here the palms are in the air and one is sitting in raised Padmasana on the buttocks.

23 Mandukasana

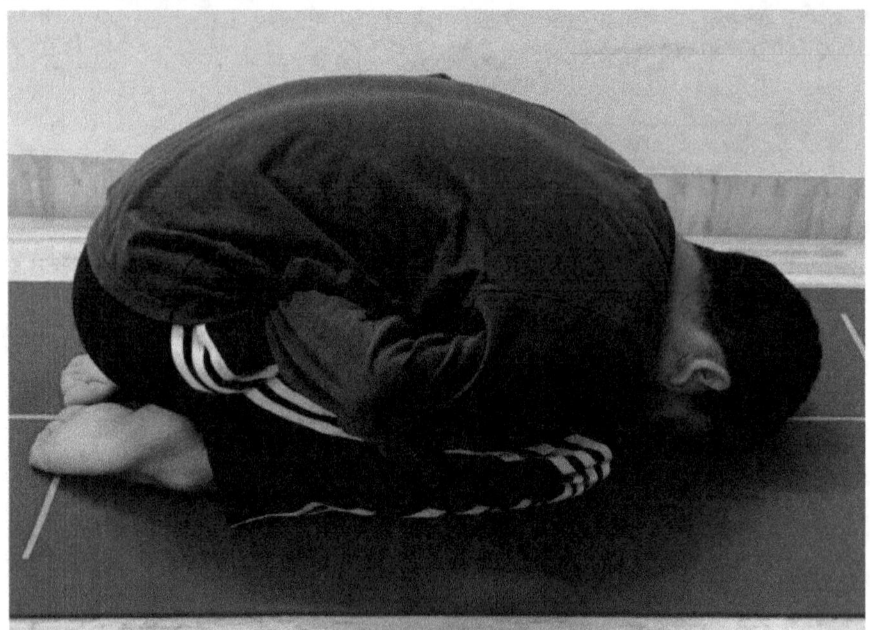

Sit in Vajrasana.
Make adi mudra of the fists.
Join the knuckles of both fists and tuck them under the belly.
Bend forward to touch the floor.

24 Uttana Mandukasana

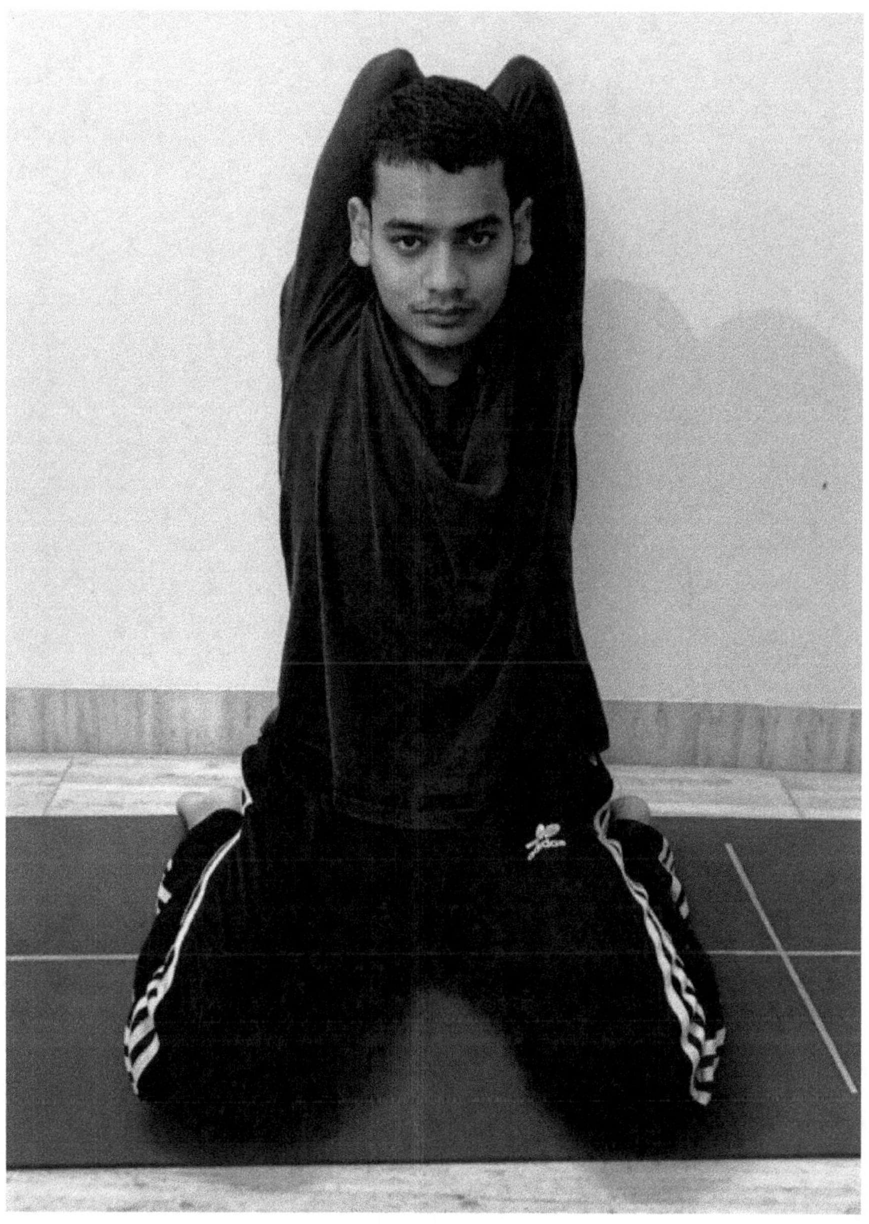

Sit like in Vajrasana, but the feet are next to the buttocks and not under. Legs are parted in a V shape. Hands behind the back on the shoulder blades. (as in third stage of Ujjayi Pranayama.)

25 Vrikshasana

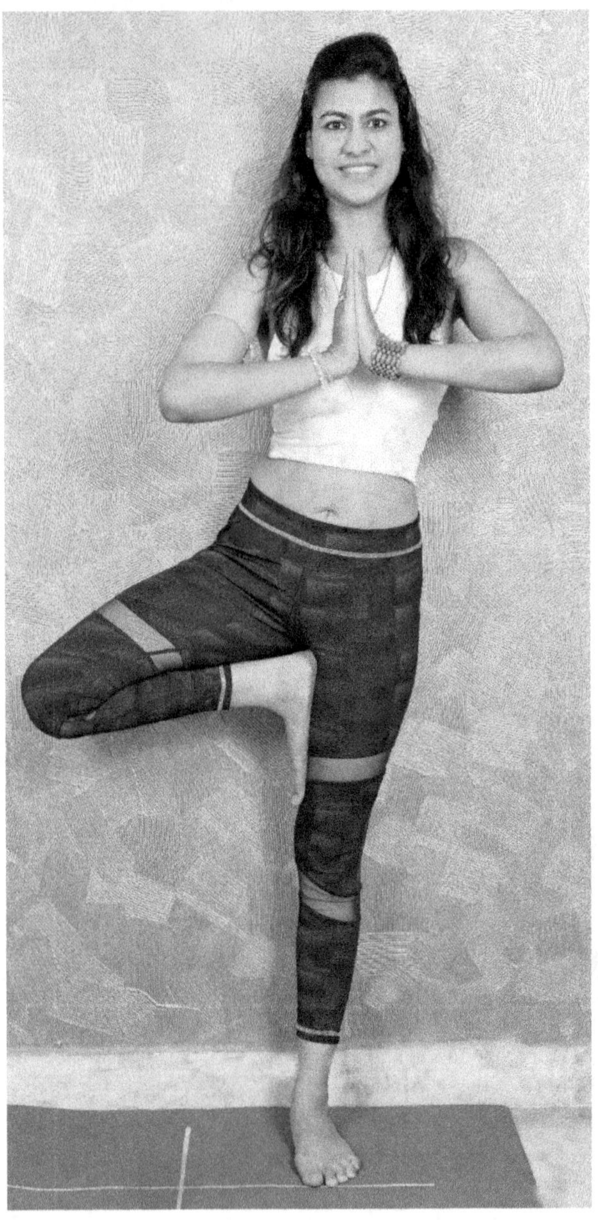

Stand with one foot firmly placed on the other thigh. Hands in Namaste or as comfortable.
Can be done with either leg on top, as comfortable.

26 Garudasana

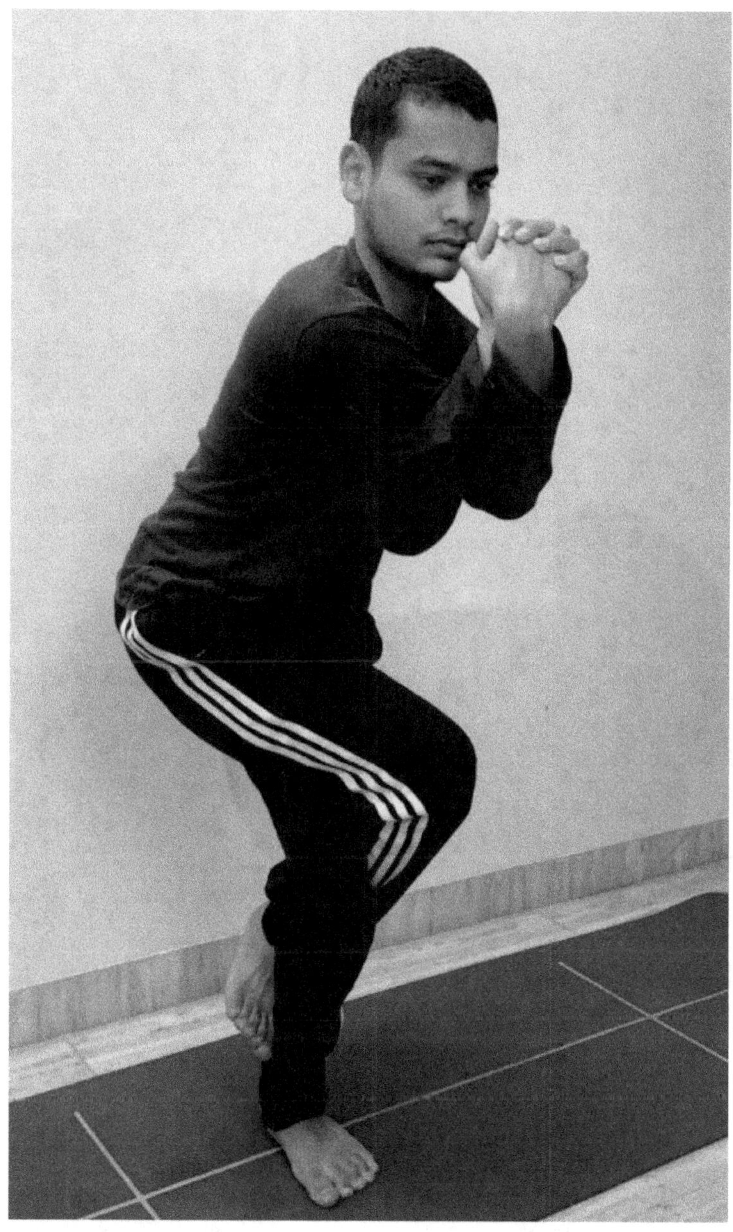

Legs are interlocked, and so are the arms. Palms firmly clasped.
Can be done with interchange of legs, as comfortable.

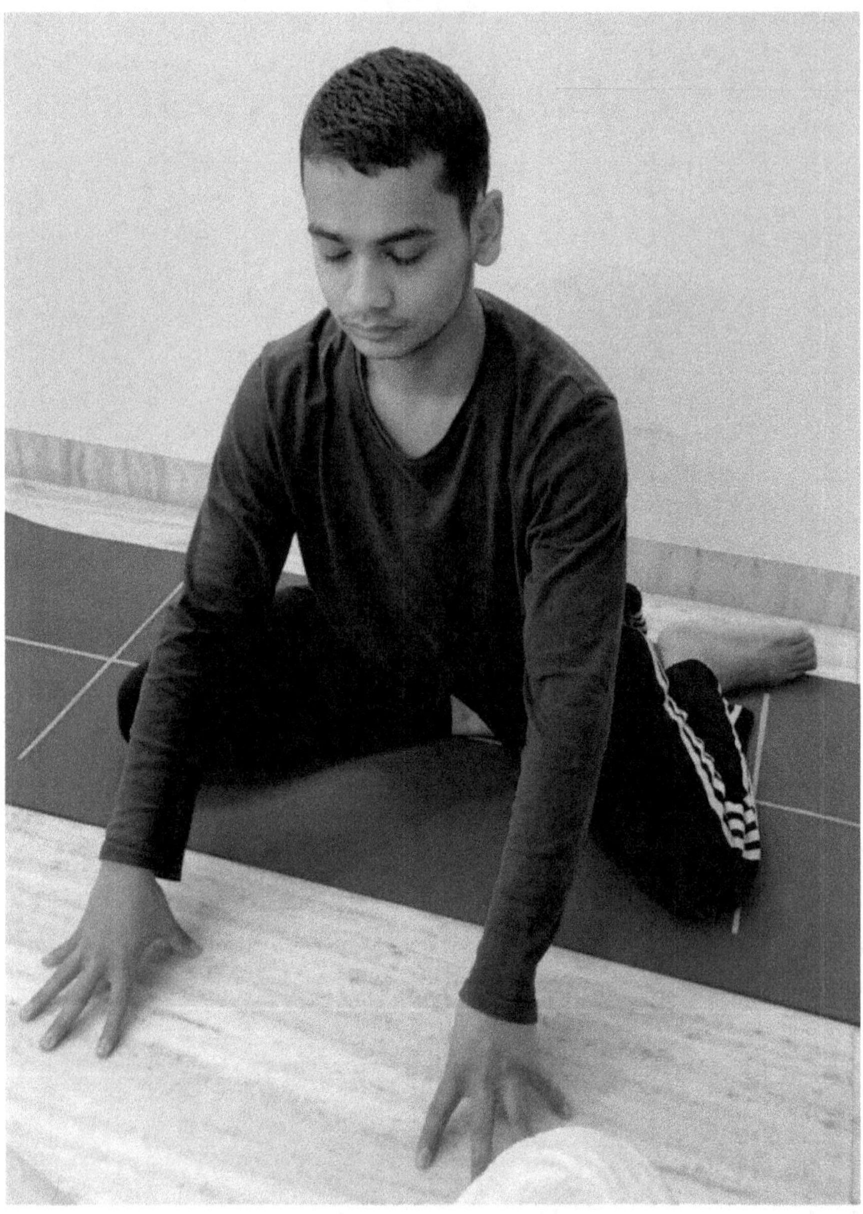

Right foot placed under the anus. Left leg folded back with left foot near the buttocks. Lunge forward to touch extended palms on the floor.

28 Shalabhasana

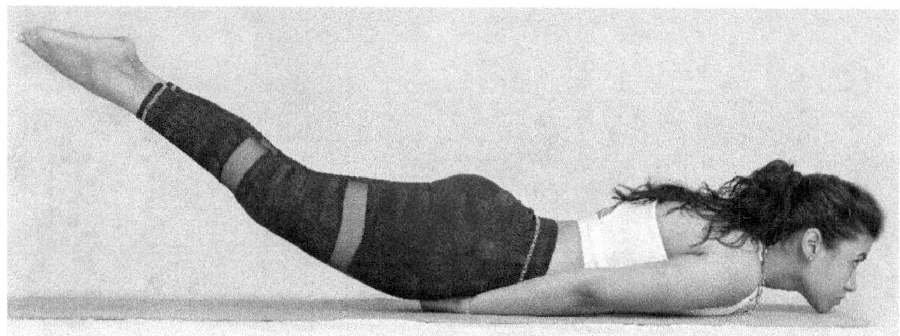

Lie down on the stomach with feet together. Make an adi mudra of the fists and place them in the groin, under the thighs. Slowly raise both legs 6" to 1 foot off the ground. (Note that this is NOT purna shalabhasana, it is simply shalabhasana with both legs. In purna shalabhasana, the legs are lifted all the way up and feet are placed on the head!)

This is actually three asanas, done with alternate legs, and with both legs.

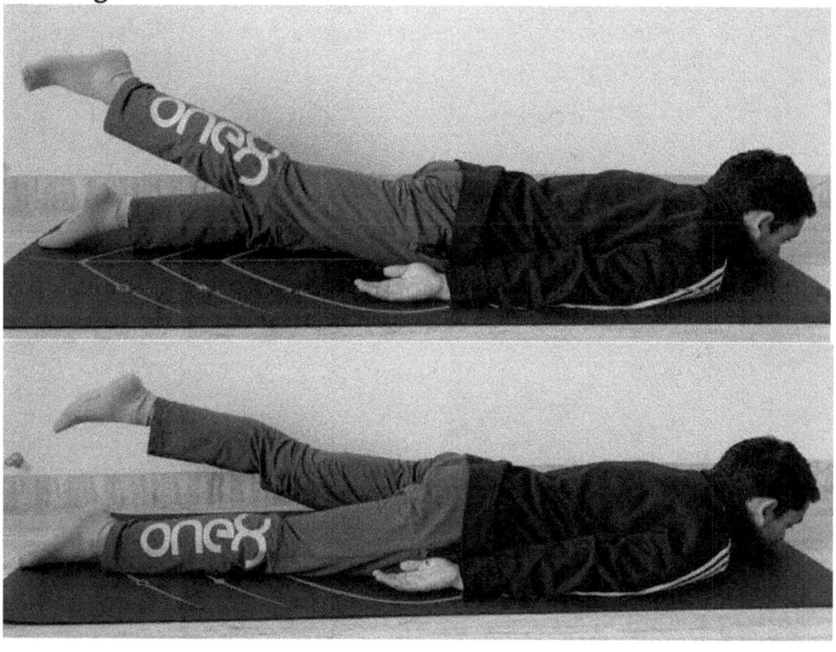

29 Makarasana

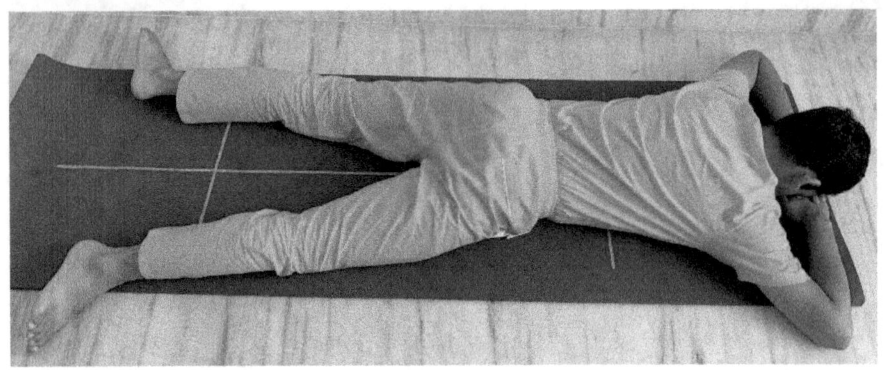

An ultimate healing pose for the spinal column.

Lie down on the stomach.
Legs outstretched with a sufficient gap.
Toes pointing away from each other.

30 Ushtrasana

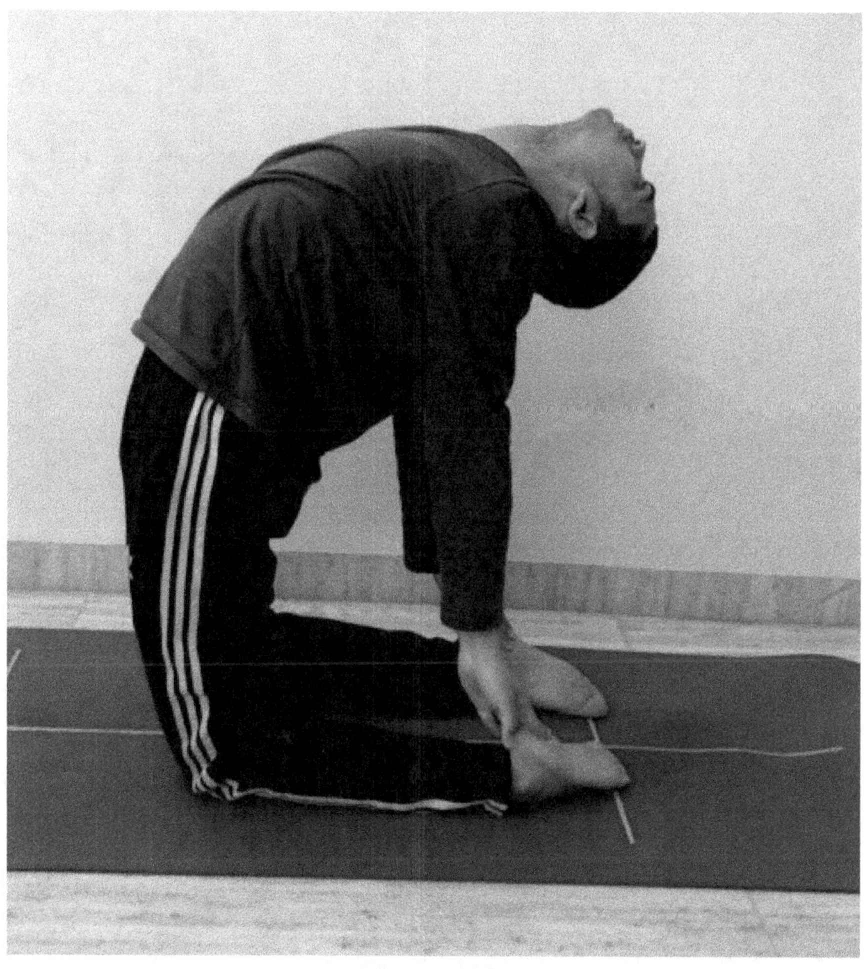

Rise up from Vajrasana and go all the way backwards, so that the hands rest on the feet.

These is a comfortable gap inbetween both legs.
Neck tilted without strain.

31 Bhujangasana

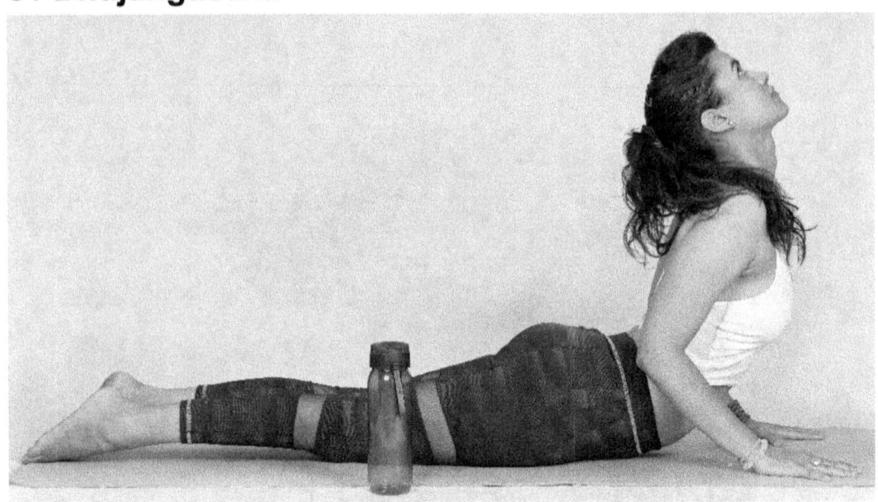

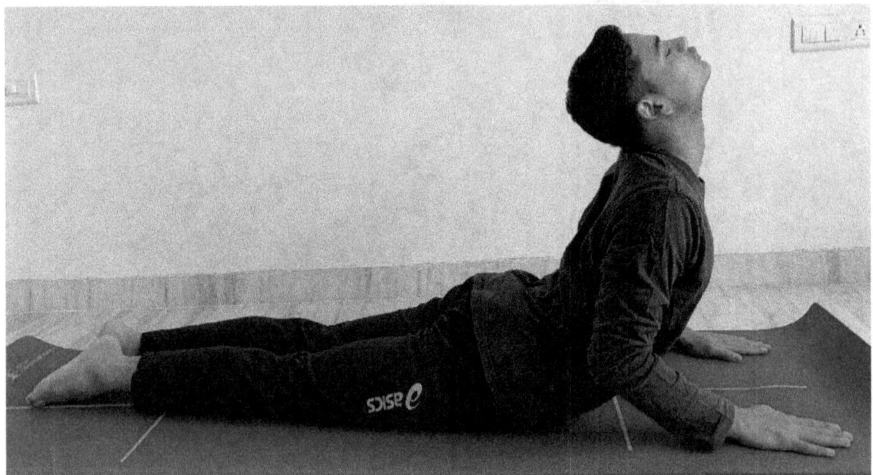

Cobra is the best asana in the Yoga Philosophy. It does whatever is needed to keep the spine healthy, and organs in the pelvis and chest well-massaged.

This is slightly different from the urdhva mukha svanasana (upward facing dog). In that posture, the legs are lifted a bit. Here the legs are touching the ground till the navel.

32 Yogasana / Ardha Padmasana

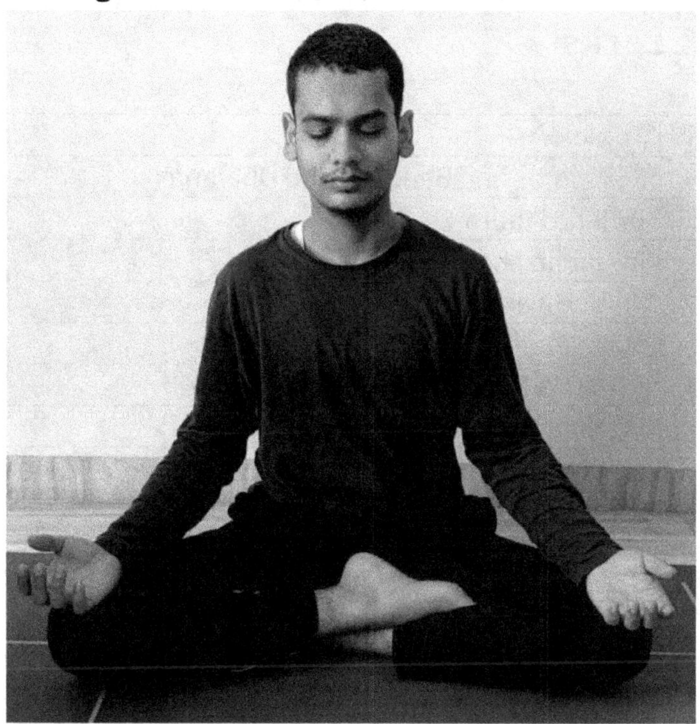

Feet position are different from Siddhasana. The toe of left foot is inside here whereas in Siddhasana it is protruding out.

It is more or less the ardha padmasana and can be done with alternate leg position by all.

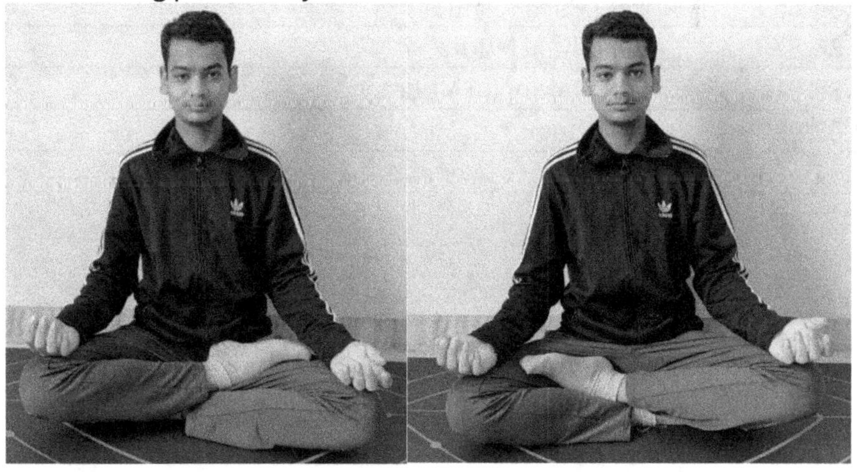

Chapter 3a – Mudra & Bandha - Twenty Types of Gestures & Locks

01 Maha Mudra

02 Nabho Mudra

03 Uddiyana Bandha

04 Jalandhar Bandha

05 Moola Bandha

06 Maha Bandha

07 Maha Vedha

08 Khechari

09 Viparitkarni

10 Yoni

11 Vajroli

12 Shaktichalani

13 Tadagi

14 Manduki

15 Shambhavi Mudra

16 Ashwini Mudra

17 Pashini Mudra

18 Kaki Mudra

19 Matangini Mudra

20 Bhujangini Mudra

Chapter 3b – Dharana – Five Types of Imagination Focus

Verse	Topic
3.68-69	25 Mudras and Bandhas and Dharanas.
3.70-71	i) Adho Dharana=Below Focus- Earth Imagination
3.72-74	ii) Ambhasi Dharana - Water Imagination
3.75-76	iii) Vaishvanari Dharana – Fire Imagination
3.77-79	iv) Vayavi Dharana – Air Imagination
3.80-81	iv) Vyoma Dharana – Space Imagination

I Adho Dharana - Earth Imagination

II Ambhasi Dharana - Water Imagination

III Vaishvanari Dharana – Fire Imagination

IV Vayavi Dharana – Air Imagination

V Vyoma Dharana – Space Imagination

Chapter 4 – Pratyahara – Five Sensory Controls

Verse	Topic
4.2	Thoughts, Memory triggers.
4.3	Sight control/awareness makes the mind Still.
4.4	Hearing and Speech / Praise or Blame Control.
4.5	Touch, Atmosphere, Body sensations awareness.
4.6	Odors and Fragrances Check.
4.7	Tongue and Taste under Check.

I Sight control makes the mind Still

II Hearing and Speech control enhances Personality

III Touch Sense restraint controls Lust

IV Odors awareness prevents infection

V Tongue & Taste restraint prevents illness and injury

Chapter 5 – Pranayama – Breath Regulation

Breath is the veritable link between the body and the mind. When we are agitated or angry, our breath has a noticeable pulsation, and when we are relaxed and happy, our breath is soft and unnoticeable.

Conversely, it is an established fact that changing the breathing pattern changes the thoughts in the mind, and has a profound effect on the body as well.

The famous Sudarshan Kriya powerful breathing technique taught in the Art of Living Happiness courses worldwide is a proven testimony and an established remedy for culturing the mind and strengthening the body by means of the Breath.

Gheranda Samhita

अथातः सम्प्रवक्ष्यामि प्राणायामस्य सद्विधिम् ।

यस्य साधनमात्रेण देवतुल्यो भवेत् नरः ॥ ५.१

athātaḥ sampravakṣyāmi prāṇāyāmasya sadvidhim |

yasya sādhanamātreṇa devatulyo bhavet naraḥ || 5.1

5.1 Now in proper and precise detail hear from me the correct method of Breath control Pranayama. Its judicious practice makes a human akin to the celestials in virtues, splendor and vitality.

Verse	Topic
5.1-2	Introduction
5.3-7	Sthanam – personal Space, place management.
5.8-15	Ritucharya – Seasonal considerations.
5.16-32	Mitahara - Food and Diet that is as per body type.
5.33-96	Breathing Techniques.
5.49-55	Nadi Shodhana
5.60-65	Prana Apana etc. 5 Vayus and 5 Upa Vayus.

5.69-72	Ujjayi Breath
5.75-77	Bhastrika count of 20 breaths with Maha Bandha, i.e Moola, Uddiyana, Jalandhara - 3 Rounds.
5.78	Brahmari or OM Chanting thrice.
5.84	Soham Breathing or Sudarshan Kriya.

No progress is possible if our diet is mainly fast food, on the run, and without a plan. This is clearly highlighted in the text in this chapter.

Gheranda Samhita

शुद्धं सु–मधुरं स्निग्धम् उदर–अर्ध–विवर्जितम् ।

भुज्यते सु–रसं प्रीत्या मित–आहारम् इमं विदुः ॥ ५.२१

śuddham su–madhuram snigdham udara–ardha–vivarjitam |

bhujyate su-rasam prītyā mita–āhāram imam viduh || 5.21

5.21 Pure and Freshly prepared,

delicious,

good for the nerves and muscles,

half-belly full

Nourishing to the soul,

inclusive of juices and soups and well cooked,

such is the diet friendly to the body and mind.

Chapter 6 – Dhyana – Three Types of Meditation by Contemplation

Verse	Topic
6.1	Introduction
6.2-8	i)Sthula Dhyana – Gross Contemplation on Deity/Guru/Favorite Image
6.9-11	Gross Contemplation on Lotus/Seed Letters/Om
6.12	Nada and Bindu with Paduka – Meditation on Two Swans and a pair of Sandals
6.13-14	Gross Contemplation on form of Guru dressed in Pure White robes.
6.15-17	ii)Jyotis Dhyana - Two types of Light Contemplation.
6.18-20	iii)Sukshama Dhyana - Subtle Vibrations Meditation.
6.21-22	Conclusion

I Sthula Dhyana – Gross Contemplation on Deity/Guru/Image

II Jyotis Dhyana - Light Contemplation

III Sukshama Dhyana - Subtle Vibrations Meditation

Chapter 7 – Samadhi – Six Types of Dissolving

I Dhyana Samadhi – Dissolve in Contemplation

II Nada Samadhi – Dissolve in Sound

III Rasananda Samadhi – Dissolve in Taste

IV Laya Samadhi – Dissolve in Touch

V Bhakti Yoga Samadhi - Dissolve in Divine Love

VI Raja Yoga Samadhi - Dissolve in Critical Analysis

Gheranda Samhita Practical Commentary

Body enjoys hard work. Good physical labor thrills the body.

A routine whereby joints and muscles are properly flexed and the breath gets worked up, brings out the best in the body. It helps immensely in maintaining body strength and flexibility, keeps the mind alert and open, and the attitude respectful and humane.

Patanjali Yoga Sutras

स्थिरसुखमासनम् ॥ २.४६ ॥ sthirasukhamāsanam ॥ 2.46 ॥

स्थिर–सुखम् आसनम् ।

2.46 Asana is that which is Stable and Comfortable

Gheranda Samhita

आसनानि समस्तानि यावन्तो जीवजन्तवः ।

चतुरशीति–लक्षाणि शिवेन कथितानि च ॥ २.१

2.1 Body Postures or Asanas are as many as there are species of insects, birds, and animals. This has been stated by the all-knowing great Lord and attested by the soul's travel through various bodies before attaining a human birth.

1 Cleansing - Shatkarma षट्कर्मशोधनं नाम प्रथमोपदेशः

अथ घटस्थयोगकथनम् । एकदा चण्डकापालिर्गत्वा घेरण्डकुट्टिरम् । प्रणम्य विनयाद्भक्त्या घेरण्डं परिपृच्छति ॥ १ ॥ atha ghaṭasthayogakathanam | ekadā caṇḍakāpālirgatvā gheraṇḍakuṭṭiram | praṇamya vinayādbhaktyā gheraṇḍam paripṛcchati ॥ 1

1.1 Once upon a time long shrouded in the folds of fathomless eternity, a valiant man dared to walk to the very center of earth. At the center lived the imperishable soul, also known as **gher-anda**, the one primal energy that pulsated simultaneously at the circumference (ghera) and the core (anda).

The one who was outwardly sensible and inwardly sensitive.

To this supreme soul gheranda, the valiant adventurer reverentially bowed.

The adventurer is named Chanda Kapali, cool-headed, effulgent-intellect and nurturing-temperament.

श्रीचण्डकापालिरुवाच । घटस्थयोगं योगेश तत्त्वज्ञानस्य कारणम् । इदानीं श्रोतुमिच्छामि योगेश्वर वद प्रभो ॥ २ ॥ śrīcaṇḍakāpāliruvāca | ghaṭasthayogaṃ yogeśa tattvajñānasya kāraṇam | idānīm śrotumicchāmi yogeśvara vada prabho ॥ 2

1.2 O Lord, please teach me the discipline of sculpting my anatomical body so that it functions to peak performance and I rise to fame in the world of men. At the same time reveal to me that deepest secret that is the essential cornerstone of Life, that which makes the heart glow with divine love, purity and bliss.

घेरण्ड उवाच । साधु साधु महाबाहो यन्मां त्वं परिपृच्छसि । कथयामि हि ते वत्स सावधानावधारय ॥ ३ ॥ gheraṇḍa uvāca | sādhu sādhu mahābāho yanmāṃ tvaṃ paripṛcchasi | kathayāmi hi te vatsa savadhānāvadhāraya sāvadhānāvadhāraya ‖ 3

1.3 The supreme soul cracked open in unbounded joy. It welcomed the brave quest with showers of blessings. Then assuming the form of a luminous sage, it spoke softly.

"I welcome your noble yearning. Surely, I shall guide, teach, and discourse upon these mighty challenges. Get ready, buckle up, and enter the institute with total focus and heightened earnestness".

नास्ति मायासमः पाशो नास्ति योगात् परं बलम् । नास्ति ज्ञानात् परो बन्धुर्नाहङ्कारात्

परो रिपुः ‖ ४ ‖ nāsti māyāsamaḥ pāśo nāsti yogāt paraṃ balam ।

nāsti jñānāt paro bandhurnāhaṅkārāt paro ripuḥ ‖ 4

1.4 Remember you shall have to keep aside all your habits, proclivities, likes and dislikes. The iron-clad armor of Maya will have to be dispensed with as it has colored your emotions with incorrect notions that appear so real.

This has covered your intellect in the garb of religious practices, rigid official procedures and formed an invisible layer on your ego or sense of possessiveness.

Slowly and methodically we shall learn the practices of Yoga, which will establish you in a strength that is broad-minded and all-encompassing.

That will in turn ground you in a wisdom that is devoid of obstacle, that rises above contentious mindsets, and that makes you harmonious with both man and nature.

अभ्यासात्कादिवर्णानि यथा शास्त्राणि बोधयेत् । तथा योगं समासाद्य तत्त्वज्ञानं च लभ्यते

‖ ५ ‖ abhyāsātkādivarṇāni yathā śāstrāṇi bodhayet । tathā yogaṃ

samāsādya tattvajñānam ca labhyate ‖ 5

1.5 It takes a good 12 years to master reading-writing-speaking by taking admission in a good school that has a focus on character building, collective social responsibility, general awareness and respect for nature and humanity.

It takes a lot of patient practice coupled with grit and determination to achieve a respectable standing in the world of men.

Similarly, for you who is desirous of loosening the fetters which are a result of unconscious impressions of countless births, a steady and aptly followed plan of mindfulness, meditation, and physical discipline shall get you home.

सुकृतैर्दुष्कृतैः कार्यैर्जायते प्राणिनां घटः । घटादुत्पद्यते कर्म घटीयन्त्रं यथा भ्रमेत् ॥ ६

sukṛtairduṣkṛtaiḥ kāryairjāyate prāṇināṃ ghaṭaḥ | ghaṭādutpadyate

karma ghaṭīyantraṃ yathā bhramet || 6

1.6 All noble deeds leave historical impressions in the world that are followed by subsequent generations. The immoral acts also serve as guides to others to avoid similar pitfalls.

History has an uncanny propensity to repeat itself. The brave souls learn therefrom and follow the wise paths.

To a distant observer these happenings appear cyclical.

ऊर्ध्वाधो भ्रमते यद्वत् घटीयन्त्रं गवां वशात् । तद्वत्कर्मवशात् जीवो भ्रमते जन्ममृत्युभिः

॥ ७ ॥ ūrdhvādho bhramate yadvat ghaṭīyantraṃ gavāṃ vaśāt |

tadvatkarmavaśāt jīvo bhramate janmamṛtyubhiḥ || 7

1.7 A wonderful imagery of bullocks drawing water from a well, and repeatedly emptying and filling the buckets is portrayed. This powerful allegory poses the ultimate question - does it all ever end? Is the movie an everlasting ordeal? is every success a prelude to a bigger challenge? Shall I find deep rest, that is blissful contented and long-lasting?

आमकुम्भ इवाम्भस्थो जीर्यमाणः सदा घटः । योगानलेन सन्दह्य घटशुद्धिं समाचरेत् ॥८

āmakumbha ivāmbhastho jīryamāṇaḥ sadā ghaṭaḥ । yogānalena

sandahya ghaṭaśuddhiṃ samācaret ॥ 8

1.8 Another powerful allegory is now presented to settle the matter decisively.

Only half-baked mud pots suffer dents, disfigurement, and disgrace. Well sculpted properly schooled and designed to be tamperproof, the yogic personalities seamlessly sport in the magnificent play, living a life that is creative, exciting, helpful, and blissful.

अथ सप्तसाधनम् । atha saptasādhanam ।

शोधनं दृढता चैव स्थैर्यं धैर्यं च लाघवम् । प्रत्यक्षं च निर्लिप्तं च घटसस्य सप्तसाधनम् ॥ ९

śodhanaṃ dṛḍhatā caiva sthairyaṃ dhairyaṃ ca lāghavam ।

pratyakṣaṃ ca nirliptaṃ ca ghaṭasasya saptasādhanam ॥ 9

1.9 The training and grounding in Yoga is a seven-fold seven-step discipline. These seven sadhanas are both concurrent and sequential. They are to be acquired simultaneously and nurtured diligently.

A) purifying the body and environment.
B) instilling determination in the intellect.
C) steadying the senses and not allowing them to stray needlessly.
D) sowing the seed of endurance in the heart, so that emotional mood-swings do not cause flutter.
E) introducing acceptance, forgiveness, and the capacity to drop and let-go, in both the mind and the heart, so that Success can come naturally.
F) strengthening awareness, discrimination, and right intention so that bliss and joy can flow.
G) becoming steeped in faith and vairagya dispassion, so that the soul remains stainless.

अथ सप्तसाधनलक्षणम् । atha saptasādhanalakṣaṇam ।

षड्कर्मणां शोधनं च आसनेन भवेद्दृढम् । मुद्रया स्थिरता चैव प्रत्याहारेण धीरता ॥ १०॥

प्राणायामाल्लाघवं च ध्यानात्प्रत्यक्षमात्मनि ।समाधिना निर्लिप्तं च मुक्तिरेव न संशयः॥११

ṣaṭkarmaṇām śodhanam ca āsanena bhaveddṛḍham | mudrayā

sthiratā caiva pratyāhāreṇa dhīratā || 10 || prāṇāyāmāllāghavam ca

dhyānātpratyakṣamātmani |samādhinā nirliptam ca muktireva na

samśayaḥ || 11

1.10-11 Body is purified by Shatkarma.
Intellect gets strong determination by Asana.
Senses are held by Mudras.
Endurance and broad vision are developed by Pratyahara.
Heart is made soft and forgiving by Pranayama.
Right awareness is the result of Meditation.
Samadhi leads to freedom from duality.

अथ शोधनम् । atha śodhanam ।

धौतिर्बस्तिस्तथा नेतिर्लौलिकी त्राटकं तथा। कपालभातिश्चैतानि षड्कर्माणि समाचरेत् ॥१२

dhautirbastistathā netirlaulikī trāṭakam tathā | kapālabhātiścaitāni

ṣaṭkarmāṇi samācaret || 12

1.12 Shatkarma consists of a) Dhauti b) Basti c) Neti d) Lauliki e)
Trataka and f) Kapalbhati
https://www.youtube.com/watch?v=WhfBD9WjlHE

Ist Shatkarma – Dhauti

अथ धौतिः । atha dhautiḥ ।

अन्तर्धौतिर्दन्तधौतिर्हृद्धौतिर्मूलशोधनम्।धौतिं चतुर्विधां कृत्वा घटं कुर्वन्ति निर्मलम् ॥ १३

antardhautirdantadhautirhṛddhautirmūlaśodhanam |

dhautim caturvidhām kṛtvā ghaṭam kurvanti nirmalam || 13

1.13 Dhauti purifies the internal organs and also established
oneness with the environment. It is of 4 types, viz cleaning the food
pipe from inside, cleaning the teeth tongue and gums, clearing the

heart, and washing the rectum.

अथ अन्तर्धौतिः । atha antardhautiḥ । वातसारं वारिसारं वह्निसारं बहिष्कृतम् । घटस्य निर्मलार्थाय अन्तर्धौतिश्चतुर्विधा ॥ १४ ॥ vātasāraṃ vārisāraṃ vahnisāraṃ bahiṣkṛtam । ghaṭasya nirmalārthāya antardhautiścaturvidhā ॥ 14

1.14 specifically for the body balancing and alignment, and also maintaining the freshness of the environment, antardhauti is of 4 types namely vatasara - by and of wind, varisara - by and of water, vahnisara - by and of fire, and bahiskrita.

अथ वातसारः । atha vātasāraḥ ।

काकचञ्चूवदास्येन पिबेद्वायुं शनैः शनैः । चालयेदुदरं पश्चाद्वर्त्मना रेचयेच्छनैः ॥ १५ kākacañcūvadāsyena pibedvāyuṃ śanaiḥ śanaiḥ । cālayedudaraṃ paścādvartmanā recayecchanaiḥ ॥ 15

1.15 vatasara helps to keep the air pure and we suck this pure air inside the belly, move it around and expel it through the anus, like passing wind.

वातसारं परं गोप्यं देहनिर्मलकारणम् । सर्वरोगक्षयकरं देहानलविवर्धकम् ॥ १६ vātasāraṃ paraṃ gopyaṃ dehanirmalakāraṇam । sarvarogakṣayakaraṃ dehānalavivardhakam ॥ 16

1.16 Vatasara is extremely difficult to learn and only the rare person can perform it effectively. It increases the digestive fire and thus burns all toxins and makes the metabolism well.

अथ वारिसारः । atha vārisāraḥ ।

आकण्ठं पूरयेद्वारि वक्त्रेण च पिबेच्छनैः । चालयेदुदरेणैव चोदराद्रेचयेदधः ॥ १७ ākaṇṭhaṃ pūrayedvāri vaktreṇa ca pibecchanaiḥ । cālayedudareṇaiva codarādrecayedadhaḥ ॥ 17

1.17 Suck water into the throat down to the belly, move it around, and urinate it out.

वारिसारं परं गोप्यं देहनिर्मलकारकम् । साधयेत् तत् प्रयत्नेन देवदेहं प्रपद्यते ॥ १८

वारिसारं परां धौतिं साधयेद्यः प्रयत्नतः । मलदेहं शोधयित्वा देवदेहं प्रपद्यते ॥ १९

vārisāraṃ paraṃ gopyaṃ dehanirmalakārakam l sādhayet tat prayatnena devadehaṃ prapadyate ‖ 18 ‖ vārisāraṃ parāṃ dhautiṃ sādhayedyaḥ prayatnataḥ l maladehaṃ śodhayitvā devadehaṃ prapadyate ‖ 19

1.18 - 19 The process is not at all understood by the average person, it needs skill to practice, and only a brilliant personality can do it effectively.

अथ अग्निसारः । atha agnisāraḥ । नाभिग्रन्थिं मेरुपृष्ठे शतवारं च कारयेत् ।

अग्निसारमेषा धौतिर्योगिनां योगसिद्धिदा ॥ २० ॥ nābhigranthiṃ merupṛṣṭhe śatavāraṃ ca kārayet lagnisārameṣā dhautiryogināṃ yogasiddhidā ‖

1.20 In Agnisara we exhale completely, and pull the empty belly to touch the spine, and pump the empty belly back and forth, and rotate its muscles as well. This is a preliminary yet significant process on the Yogic path. It raises the digestive fire, this burns away toxins and undigested food, thoughts and emotions.

https://www.youtube.com/watch?v=BVfOKvsvf9o

उदरामयजं त्यक्त्वा जठराग्निं विवर्धयेत् । एषा धौतिः परा गोप्या देवानामपि दुर्लभा ।

केवलं धौतिमात्रेण देवदेहो भवेद् ध्रुवम् ॥ २१ ॥ udarāmayajaṃ tyaktvā jaṭharāgniṃ vivardhayet l eṣā dhautiḥ parā gopyā devānāmapi durlabhā l kevalaṃ dhautimātreṇa devadeho bhaved dhruvam ‖ 21

1.21 again this practice can only be done by a strong determination, it cannot be forced on anyone, since the desire to do it should come from within. It has been observed that only the most intelligent perform it correctly.

अथ बहिष्कृतधौतिः । atha bahiṣkṛtadhautiḥ । काकीमुद्रां साधयित्वा पूरयेदुदरं मरुत् । धारयेदर्द्धयामं तु चालयेदधोवर्त्मना । एषा धौतिः परा गोप्या न प्रकाश्या कदाचन ॥ २२ ॥ dhārayedarddhayāmaṃ tu cālayedadhovartmanā । eṣā dhautiḥ parā gopyā na prakāśyā kadācana ॥ 22

1.22 A rare practice is the bahiskrita Dhauti, or intestinal cleansing by sucking air down through the belly to the small intestine, where by slow peristalsis it helps dislodge crumbs stuck in the pores. Scrubs away all undigested food particles, and increases the efficacy of intestine.

अथ प्रक्षालनम् । atha prakṣālanam । नाभिमग्नजले स्थित्वा शक्तिनाडीं विसर्जयेत् । कराभ्यां क्षालयेन्नाडीं यावन्मलविसर्जनम् । तावत्प्रक्षाल्य नाडीं च उदरे वेशयेत्पुनः ॥ २३

nābhimagnajale sthitvā śaktināḍīṃ visarjayet । karābhyāṃ kṣālayennāḍīṃ yāvanmalavisarjanam । tāvatprakṣālya nāḍīṃ ca udare veśayetpunaḥ ॥ 23

1.23 Laghu Shankh Prakshalanam needs the crow walk to help circulate lukewarm salt water all through the stomach, duodenum, small intestine and colon. The whole process should take 90 minutes. One may gulp lukewarm saltwater, walk few meters in crow walk, and whenever pressure is felt go to the toilet. Repeat this sequence enough times until one sees clear fluid emanating out of the anus, however stop the process after 45 minutes, then lie down covered by a blanket and take complete rest for 45 minutes.

इदं प्रक्षालनं गोप्यं देवानामपि दुर्लभम् । केवलं धौतिमात्रेण देवदेहो भवेद्ध्रुवम् ॥ २४

idaṃ prakṣālanam gopyaṃ devānāmapi durlabham । kevalaṃ dhautimātreṇa devadeho bhaveddhruvam ॥ 24

1.24 This practice must be done in seclusion without interruption, chatting, or distraction.

अथ बहिष्कृतधौतिप्रयोगः । atha bahiṣkṛtadhautiprayogaḥ ।
यामार्धं धारणां शक्ति यावन्न साधयेन्नरः । बहिष्कृतं महद्धौतिस्तावच्चैव न जायते ॥ २५

yāmārdhaṃ dhāraṇāṃ śaktiṃ yāvanna sādhayennaraḥ | bahiṣkṛtaṃ

mahaddhautistāvaccaiva na jāyate || 25

1.25 It must be done by people who are relatively fit in mind and body, only once a year, and ensuring the correct sequence of 90 minutes.

अथ दन्तधौतिः । atha dantadhautiḥ |

दन्तमूलं जिह्वामूलं रन्ध्रं च कर्णयुग्मयोः । कपालरन्ध्रं पञ्चैते दन्तधौतिं विधीयते ॥ २६

dantamūlaṃ jihvāmūlaṃ randhraṃ ca karṇayugmayoḥ |

kapālarandhraṃ pañcaite dantadhautiṃ vidhīyate || 26

1.26 In Cleansing of the 5 Senses, the teeth and tongue, the twin ear lobes, and pituitary gland at the forehead should be first attended to. Powder of Acacia Catechu commonly known as Khair or Khadir helps in oral hygiene. High degree of tooth, gum, and throat fitness can be achieved, and mouth illnesses cured by rubbing khadir powder on teeth and gums and tongue, or sucking khadiradi vati tablets.

https://www.1mg.com/hi/patanjali/khadir-benefits-in-hindi/

Further the text adds that rubbing manjan or toothpowder is a wonderful oral hygiene practice, as the sensations from our finger interact with the emotions sitting on our teeth and gums, and cause tremendous healing.

A daily morning and nighttime ritual for 10 minutes is recommended. The sequence is to apply and massage toothpowder (or a natural herbal toothpaste), leave it for 8-10 minutes so that enough saliva has accumulated. Then brush the teeth thoroughly and also scrub the tongue. Finally rinse well in running water. Such a technique is approved for and by Yoga practitioners.

अथ दन्तमूलधौतिः । atha dantamūladhautiḥ । gums / root of teeth cleaning ॥ खादिरेण रसेनाथ मृत्तिकया च शुद्धया । मार्जयेद्दन्तमूलं च यावत्किल्बिषमाहरेत् ॥ २७॥ दन्तमूलं परा धौतिर्योगिनां योगसाधने । नित्यं कुर्यात्प्रभाते च दन्तरक्षां च योगवित् । दन्तमूलं धावनादिकार्येषु योगिनां मतम् ॥ २८॥

अथ जिह्वाशोधनम् । atha jihvāśodhanam । cleaning the tongue ॥ अथातः संप्रवक्ष्यामि जिह्वाशोधनकारणम् । जरामरणरोगादीन्नाशयेद्दीर्घलम्बिका ॥ २९

अथ जिह्वामूलधौतिप्रयोगः । atha jihvāmūladhautiprayogaḥ । Scraping the rear of the tongue ॥ तर्जनीमध्यमानामा अङ्गुलित्रययोगतः । वेशयेद्गलमध्ये तु मार्जयेल्लम्बिकामूलम् । शनैः शनैर्मार्जयित्वा कफदोषं निवारयेत् ॥ ३० मार्जयेन्नवनीतेन दोहयेच्च पुनः पुनः । तदग्रं लोहयन्त्रेण कर्षयित्वा शनैः शनैः ॥ ३१ नित्यं कुर्यात्प्रयत्नेन रवेरुदयकेऽस्तके । एवं कृते च नित्यं सा लम्बिका दीर्घतां व्रजेत् ॥३२

khādireṇa rasenātha mṛttikayā ca śuddhayā । mārjayeddantamūlaṃ ca yāvatkilbiṣamāharet ॥ 27 ॥ dantamūlaṃ parā dhautiryoginām yogasādhane । nityaṃ kuryātprabhāte ca dantarakṣāṃ ca yogavit । dantamūlaṃ dhāvanādikāryeṣu yoginām matam ॥ 28 ॥ athātaḥ sampravakṣyāmi jihvāśodhanakāraṇam । arāmaraṇarogādīnnāśayeddīrghalambikā ॥ 29 tarjanīmadhyamānāmā aṅgulitrayayogataḥ । veśayedgalamadhye tu mārjayellambikāmūlam । śanaiḥ śanairmārjayitvā kaphadoṣaṃ nivārayet ॥ 30 ॥ mārjayennavanītena dohayecca punaḥ punaḥ । tadagraṃ lohayantreṇa karṣayitvā śanaiḥ śanaiḥ ॥ 31 ॥ nityaṃ kuryātprayatnena raverudayake'stake । evaṃ kṛte ca nityaṃ sā lambikā dīrghatāṃ vrajet ॥ 32

1.27-32 now the method of gums and tongue cleaning is described. A regular massage of the tongue with the three fingers greatly helps in proper saliva production, in making speech soft and unharmful, and improving the taste buds. Whereby many illnesses caused by eating rotten, insipid, improperly cooked food can be prevented. Life can be lengthened by the increased production of saliva that goes inside with the breath and makes the lungs and heart very strong. Untimely death can be prevented due to soft speech that does not arouse rage in opponents.

Such regular care morning and evening removes all pent-up emotions and thereby ensures freshness in body and mind.

अथ कर्णधौतिप्रयोगः । atha karṇadhautiprayogaḥ । ear cleaning

तर्जन्यनामिकायोगान्मार्जयेत् कर्णरन्ध्रयोः ।नित्यमभ्यासयोगेन नादान्तरं प्रकाशयेत् ॥३३

tarjanyanāmikāyogānmārjayet karṇarandhrayoḥ |

nityamabhyāsayogena nādāntaraṃ prakāśayet || 33

1.33 Ears are highly susceptible to catching angry and bitter and harmful sounds, so the index finger or ring finger may be employed to massage the ear lobes. This will trigger the protective muscle that keeps the hurtful noises minimum. Moreover it shall increase the receptivity of ears towards the divine frequencies and produce blissful tendencies.

अथ कपालरन्ध्रप्रयोगः । atha kapālarandhraprayogaḥ । sinuses

वृद्धाङ्गुष्ठेन दक्षेण मार्जयेद्भालरन्ध्रकम् । एवमभ्यासयोगेन कफदोषं निवारयेत् ॥ ३४

vṛddhāṅguṣṭhena dakṣeṇa mārjayedbhālarandhrakam |

evamabhyāsayogena kaphadoṣaṃ nivārayet || 34

1.34 The frontal lobes of the brain and sinuses are to be kept active by massage with thumb and fingertip at the depressions at template, third eye, and around the eyes.

This keeps all glands clean and healthy. illnesses that occur every two months at weather change are thus prevented.

नाडी निर्मलतां याति दिव्यदृष्टिः प्रजायते। निद्रान्ते भोजनान्ते च दिवान्ते च दिने दिने॥३५

nāḍī nirmalatāṃ yāti divyadṛṣṭiḥ prajāyate| nidrānte bhojanānte ca

divānte ca dine dine || 35

1.35 Intuition develops when endocrine system is in robust health since the glands are directly affecting chakras. The physiological alignment keeps the nerves happy and the energy of the individual remains high.

This massage of the sinuses and face marma can be done two three times a day.

अथ हृद्धौतिः । atha hṛddhautiḥ । हृद्धौतिं त्रिविधां कुर्याद्दण्डवमनवाससा ॥ ३६

hṛddhautiṃ trividhāṃ kuryāddaṇḍavamanavāsasā ॥ 36

1.36 Digestive system (or emotions of heart) cleansing is of 3 kinds. By means of a stick, or by vomiting or by means of a cloth. That is to say that hate is to be kept out by a stick, fear by vomiting out, and love to be kindled by a soft cloth.

अथ दण्डहृद्धौतिः । atha daṇḍahṛddhautiḥ ।

रम्भादण्डं हरिद्दण्डं वेत्रदण्डं तथैव च । हृन्मध्ये चालयित्वा तु पुनः प्रत्याहरेच्छनैः ॥ ३७

rambhādaṇḍam hariddaṇḍam vetradaṇḍam tathaiva ca ।

hṛnmadhye cālayitvā tu punaḥ pratyāharecchanaiḥ ॥ 37

1.37 A suitable soft smooth rubbery stick is slowly inserted into the throat and rotated to clean the esophagus.

कफपित्तं तथा क्लेदं रेचयेदूर्ध्ववर्त्मना । दण्डधौतिविधानेन हृद्रोगं नाशयेद्ध्रुवम् ॥ ३८

kaphapittam tathā kledam recayedūrdhvavartmanā ।

daṇḍadhautividhānena hṛdrogam nāśayeddhruvam ॥ 38

1.38 It scrubs away remnants of food, phlegm, bile and digestive fluids and thus causes hate to depart from the heart.

अथ वमनधौतिः । atha vamanadhautiḥ । भोजनान्ते पिबेद्वारि चाकण्ठपूरितं सुधीः । ऊर्ध्वां दृष्टिं क्षणं कृत्वा तज्जलं वमयेत्पुनः । नित्यमभ्यासयोगेन कफपित्तं निवारयेत् ॥

३९ ॥ bhojanānte pibedvāri cākaṇṭhapūritaṃ sudhīḥ । ūrdhvāṃ

dṛṣṭiṃ kṣaṇaṃ kṛtvā tajjalaṃ vamayetpunaḥ ।

nityamabhyāsayogena kaphapittaṃ nivārayet ॥ 39

1.39 Directly after a meal, drink water and continue drinking until vomiting sensation occurs, then vomit it all out.

Doing it a few times over a week banishes fear that is the cause of undigested phlegm and bile, otherwise known in Ayurveda as Kapha and Pitta dosha.

अथ वासोधौतिः । atha vāsodhautiḥ ।

चतुरङ्गुलविस्तारं सूक्ष्मवस्त्रं शनैर्ग्रसेत् । पुनः प्रत्याहरेदेतत्प्रोच्यते धौतिकर्मकम् ॥ ४०

गुल्मज्वरप्लीहाकुष्ठकफपित्तं विनश्यति । आरोग्यं बलपुष्टिश्च भवेत्तस्य दिने दिने ॥ ४१

caturaṅgulavistāraṃ sūkṣmavastraṃ śanairgraset । punaḥ

pratyāharedetatprocyate dhautikarmakam ॥ 40

gulmajvaraplīhākuṣṭhakaphapittaṃ vinaśyati । ārogyaṃ balapuṣṭiśca

bhavettasya dine dine ॥ 41

1.40- 41 Slowly swallow a 4-inch-wide soft thin cotton cloth that is a few feet long, then slowly pull it out. It shall reach deep into the innards and release all pent up emotions, undigested thoughts, broken promises, and make love blossom again.

https://www.youtube.com/watch?v=ob5FtphCbCk

अथ मूलशोधनम् । atha mūlaśodhanam । colon cleaning

अपानक्रूरता तावद्यावन्मूलं न शोधयेत् । तस्मात्सर्वप्रयत्नेन मूलशोधनमाचरेत् ॥ ४२

apānakrūratā tāvadyāvanmūlaṃ na śodhayet ।

tasmātsarvaprayatnena mūlaśodhanamācaret ॥ 42

1.42 Apana vayu that is so important for excretion and also disconnection from the body-mind complex for deep rest and meditation, can never function fully if the colon is weak or unclean.

पीतमूलस्य दण्डेन मध्यमाङ्गुलिनाऽपि वा । यत्नेन क्षालयेद्गुह्यं वारिणा च पुनः पुनः ॥ ४३

pītamūlasya daṇḍena madhyamāṅgulinā'pi vā । yatnena

kṣālayedguhyaṃ vāriṇā ca punaḥ punaḥ ॥ 43

1.43 a naturopathy practice of colon cleansing - enema can be followed once in few years to make the colon strong and healthy.

वारयेत्कोष्ठकाठिन्यमामजीर्णं निवारयेत् । कारणं कान्तिपुष्ट्योश्च वह्निमण्डलदीपनम् ॥४४

vārayetkoṣṭhakāṭhinyamāmajīrṇaṃ nivārayet | kāraṇaṃ

kāntipuṣṭhyośca vahnimaṇḍaladīpanam || 44

1.44 This relieves one from all types of stored up and stuffed up indigestion and Indigestive tendency.
As digestion improves and metabolism becomes normal, beauty returns to the skin, the face glows, and stamina gets enhanced.

IInd Shatkarma Basti

अथ बस्तिप्रकरणम् । atha bastiprakaraṇam । जलबस्तिः शुष्कबस्तिर्बस्तिः स्याद् द्विविधा स्मृता । जलबस्तिं जले कुर्याच्छुष्कबस्तिं सदा क्षितौ ॥ ४५

jalabastiḥ śuṣkabastirbastiḥ syād dvividhā smṛtā | jalabastiṃ jale

kuryācchuṣkabastiṃ sadā kṣitau || 45

1.45 Basti purification is now described. It is of 2 types, wet and dry.

अथ जलबस्तिः । atha jalabastiḥ ।

नाभिमग्नजले पायुं न्यस्तवानुत्कटासनम् । आकुञ्चनं प्रसारं च जलबस्तिं समाचरेत् ॥ ४६

nābhimagnajale pāyuṃ nyastavānutkaṭāsanam | ākuñcanaṃ

prasāraṃ ca jalabastiṃ samācaret || 46

1.46 Drink sufficient lukewarm water and sit in Utkatasana. Then contract and dilate the anal sphincter muscles. This practice is called jala basti or wet cleansing.

प्रमेहं च उदावर्तं क्रूरवायुं निवारयेत् । भवेत्स्वच्छन्ददेहश्च कामदेवसमो भवेत् ॥ ४७

pramehaṃ ca udāvartaṃ krūravāyuṃ nivārayet |

bhavetsvacchandadehaśca kāmadevasamo bhavet || 47

1.47 this cures prameha, udavarta and krurvayu. Body gets relief from various illnesses. The face regains ruddiness and comeliness as of a celestial.

अथ शुष्कबस्तिः । atha śuṣkabastiḥ । बस्तिं पश्चिमोत्तानेन चालयित्वा शनैरधः ।
अश्विनीमुद्रया पायुमाकुञ्चयेत् प्रसारयेत् ॥ ४८ ॥ bastiṃ paścimottānena

cālayitvā śanairadhaḥ | aśvinīmudrayā pāyumākuñcayet prasārayet ‖ 48

1.48 Sit in Paschimottanasan and apply ashwini mudra. Focus on the abdomen and start contracting and dilating the anal sphincter muscles.

एवमभ्यासयोगेन कोष्ठदोषो न विद्यते । विवर्द्धयेज्जठराग्निमामवातं विनाशयेत् ॥ ४९

evamabhyāsayogena koṣṭhadoṣo na vidyate |

vivarddhayejjaṭharāgnimāmavātaṃ vināśayet ‖ 49

1.49 Constipation bids adieu, the capacity to stand firm in times of disgrace and shame and face difficult situations with elan sprouts, hypocrisy and flatulence are banished.

IIIrd Shatkarma - Sutra Neti

अथ नेतियोगः । atha netiyogaḥ | वितस्तिमानं सूक्ष्मसूत्रं नासानाले प्रवेशयेत् । मुखान्निर्गमयेत्पश्चात्प्रोच्यते नेतिकर्मकम् ॥५०॥ vitastimānaṃ sūkṣmasūtraṃ

nāsānāle praveśayet | mukhānnirgamayetpaścātprocyate

netikarmakam ‖ 50

1.50 Sutra Neti is done by passing a 3mm smooth rubber tube or cotton thread through one nostril and giving it a U-turn bringing it out from the other nostril.
https://www.youtube.com/watch?v=yoRGo2nl8ic

साधनान्नेतिकार्यस्य खेचरीसिद्धिमाप्नुयात् । कफदोषा विनश्यन्ति दिव्यदृष्टिः प्रजायते ॥५१

sādhanānnetikāryasya khecarīsiddhimāpnuyāt | kaphadoṣā

vinaśyanti divyadṛṣṭiḥ prajāyate ‖ 51

1.51 Sutra neti shatkarma develops intuition by making the sinuses healthy. Develops kechari Siddhi or kundalini shakti whereby one's bodily functions proceed at peak performance.

IVth Shatkarma - Lauliki (Nauli)

अथ लौलिकीयोगः । atha laulikīyogaḥ ।

अमन्दवेगेन तुन्दं तु भ्रामयेदुभपार्श्वयोः । सर्वरोगान्निहन्तीह देहानलविवर्द्धनम् ॥ ५२

amandavegena tundaṃ tu bhrāmayedubhapārśvayoḥ ।

sarvarogānnihantīha dehānalavivarddhanam ॥ 52

1.52 Focus on the Manipura, exhale and apply Uddiyana bandha and vigorously move the stomach and abdomen muscles up and to left and right.

https://www.easyayurveda.com/2017/12/10/nauli-karma-right-method-types-benefits/

Nauli or Lauliki Shatkarma raises the digestive fire, thus clears all undigested thoughts, burns down deep-rooted emotions and improves metabolic activity.

Vth Shatkarma – Trataka

अथ त्राटकम् । atha trāṭakam । निमेषोन्मेषकं त्यक्त्वा सूक्ष्मलक्ष्यं निरीक्षयेत् ।

यावदश्रूणि पतन्ति त्राटकं प्रोच्यते बुधैः ॥ ५३ ॥ nimeṣonmeṣakaṃ tyaktvā

sūkṣmalakṣyaṃ nirīkṣayet । yāvadaśrūṇi patanti trāṭakaṃ procyate

budhaiḥ ॥ 53

1.53 Gaze unblinkingly at a steady flame kept at eye level. for 3minutes, blink once and continue for another 2min. Tears will come, gently close the eyes. With closed eyes, do palming for another 5 minutes, taking care hands are not touching eyelids, and eye balls are free to move. Then lie down for 10minutes keeping cool Rosewater tissues over the eyes, listen to soft music.
https://www.easyayurveda.com/2019/12/17/shambhavi-mudra/

एवमभ्यासयोगेन शाम्भवी जायते ध्रुवम् । नेत्ररोगा विनश्यन्ति दिव्यदृष्टिः प्रजायते ॥ ५४

evamabhyāsayogena śāmbhavī jāyate dhruvam । netrarogā

vinaśyanti divyadṛṣṭiḥ prajāyate ॥ 54

1.54 This practice helps make bright the physical as well as the spiritual vision.
Helps going deep in meditation, i.e. Shambhavi siddhi or Shiva Shakti, whereby one's spiritual practices become well grounded.

VIth Shatkarma Kapalbhati

अथ कपालभातिः । atha kapālabhātiḥ । वातक्रमेण व्युत्क्रमेण शीत्क्रमेण विशेषतः । भालभाति त्रिधा कुर्यात्कफदोषं निवारयेत्॥५५ ॥ vātakrameṇa vyutkrameṇa śītkrameṇa viśeṣataḥ | bhālabhātiṁ tridhā kuryātkaphadoṣaṁ nivārayet || 55

1.55 Kapalbhati is of 3 types Vata-Vyut-Sheet.
All afflictions related to kapha dosha i.e. phlegm is vanquished.

अथ वातक्रमकपालभातिः । atha vātakramakapālabhātiḥ |
इडया पूरयेद्वायुं रेचयेत्पिङ्गलां पुनः । पिङ्गलया पूरयित्वा पुनश्चन्द्रेण रेचयेत् ॥ ५६
पूरकं रेचकं कृत्वा वेगेन न तु धारयेत् । एवमभ्यासयोगेन कफदोषं निवारयेत् ॥ ५७
iḍayā pūrayedvāyuṁ recayetpiṅgalāṁ punaḥ | piṅgalayā pūrayitvā punaścandreṇa recayet || 56 || pūrakaṁ recakaṁ kṛtvā vegena na tu dhārayet | evamabhyāsayogena kaphadoṣaṁ nivārayet || 57
1.56-57 Vata-kapalbhati
Alternate nostril breathing without breath retention. Begin from left nostril. Make the breath soft, silent, smooth.
It will easily balance the kapha-phlegm.

अथ व्युत्क्रमकपालभातिः । atha vyutkramakapālabhātiḥ |
नासाभ्यां जलमाकृष्य पुनर्वक्त्रेण रेचयेत्। पायं पायं व्युत्क्रमेण श्लेष्मदोषं निवारयेत् ॥५८
nāsābhyāṁ jalamākṛṣya punarvaktreṇa recayet| pāyaṁ pāyaṁ vyutkrameṇa śleṣmadoṣaṁ nivārayet || 58
1.58 Vyut-kapalbhati
Jal neti using a neti-pot having a long snout. Apply ghee to both

nostrils. Use lukewarm water, begin from left nostril and let it come out from right nostril. Reverse by refilling the jal-neti-pot.

Do few rounds of Bhastrika, clean the nose with hanky, and sit in meditation for few minutes, covered with a shawl.

अथ शीत्क्रमकपालभातिः । atha śītkramakapālabhātiḥ ।
शीत्कृत्य पीत्वा वक्त्रेण नासानालैर्विरेचयेत्। एवमभ्यासयोगेन कामदेवसमो भवेत्॥ ५९
śītkṛtya pītvā vaktreṇa nāsānālairvirecayet। evamabhyāsayogena

kāmadevasamo bhavet॥ 59
1.59 Sheet-kapalbhati
A process of gulping lukewarm water through the mouth and expelling it through the nostrils.
https://www.yogicwayoflife.com/sheetkrama-kapalbhati/

न जायते वार्द्धकं च ज्वरो नैव प्रजायते । भवेत्स्वच्छन्ददेहश्च कफदोषं निवारयेत् ॥ ६०
na jāyate vārddhakaṃ ca jvaro naiva prajāyate ।

bhavetsvacchandadehaśca kaphadoṣaṃ nivārayet ॥ 60
1.60 Benefits of Shatkarma Practice
a) senses and joints remain functional till the end
b) face wrinkles and hair loss is prevented
c) organs and tissues maintain their health as the energies related to kapha-phlegm remain in balance

॥ इति श्रीघेरण्डसंहितायां महर्षिघेरण्डनृपचण्डकापालिसंवादे घटस्थयोगे षड्कर्मशोधनं नाम प्रथमोपदेशः समाप्तः ॥ iti śrīgheraṇḍasaṃhitāyāṃ

maharṣigheraṇḍanṛpacaṇḍakāpālisaṃvāde ghaṭasthayoge

ṣaṭkarmaśodhanaṃ nāma prathamopadeśaḥ samāptaḥ ॥ Thus ends the 1st chapter

2 Posture - Asana घटस्थयोगे द्वात्रिंशासनवर्णनम्

घेरण्ड उवाच । gheraṇḍa uvāca । अभ्यासाद्यस्य देहेऽयं योगौपयिकतां व्रजेत् । मनश्च स्थिरतामेति प्रोच्यते तदिहाऽऽसनम् ॥ १ ॥ abhyāsādyasya dehe'yaṃ yogaupayikatāṃ vrajet । manaśca sthiratāmeti procyate tadihā''sanam ॥ 1

2.1 There are as many theoretical Postures of the Body as there are Bird, Animal and Insect species on the planet. These are stated to be 84 hundred thousand in number and are said to be auspicious as all living beings are created by the Divine will.

आसनानि समस्तानि यावन्तो जीवजन्तवः । चतुरशीतिलक्षाणि शिवेन कथितानि च ॥ २ āsanāni samastāni yāvanto jīvajantavaḥ । caturaśītilakṣāṇi śivena kathitāni ca ॥ 2

2.2 Out of these theoretical postures, sixteen less than a hundred (i.e. 84) are specifically conducive for mankind. These 84 asanas are especially good to do while learning, they firm up all areas of the anatomy. However, we shall enumerate only 32 Asanas since they form a complete set that can be done with regularity when out of the learning phase.

Just as 32 teeth form a complete dental structure, that can properly process all types of food. So, 32 Asanas have been enumerated as a complete set, those make the body ready to properly face all challenges encountered in a lifetime.

Here 32=8x4. A day is made up of 24 hours=8x3, and a single set of 8 hours (known as a prahar in Sanskrit) is necessary for optimal work, sleep, and entertainment.

Asanas have been mentioned as 32 or 8x4, which means that we must continue to live another set of 8 hours in another plane, after having lived wisely balancing work, rest and play. Living beyond death is the quality one attains when one balances a complete set of Postures in this life. Complete set also refers to a broad vision, being open-minded in the intellect and expansive in the heart.

As we see each Asana in detail, we realize that the physical posture cannot really be done by a mind that is averse to take on varied roles in society.

Unless at home we can play the part of a father, brother, son, spouse, engineer, nurse, architect, maid, or other varied roles, one cannot face the world at large. These asanas judiciously portray various emotions, animal traits and skills that are needed to rise in the world of men.

तेषां मध्ये विशिष्टानि षोडशोनं शतं कृतम् । तेषां मध्ये मर्त्यलोके द्वात्रिंशदासनं शुभम्॥३
सिद्धं पद्मं तथा भद्रं मुक्तं वज्रं च स्वस्तिकम् । सिंहं च गोमुखं वीरं धनुरासनमेव च ॥ ४
मृतं गुप्तं तथा मात्स्यं मत्स्येन्द्रासनमेव च । गोरक्षं पश्चिमोत्तानमुत्कटं सङ्कटं तथा ॥ ५
मयूरं कुक्कुटं कूर्मं तथा चोत्तानकूर्मकम् । उत्तानमण्डूकं वृक्षं मण्डूकं गरुडं वृषम् ॥ ६
शलभं मकरं चोष्ट्रं भुजङ्गं च योगासनम् । द्वात्रिंशदासनानि तु मर्त्यलोके हि सिद्धिदम् ॥ ७

teṣāṃ madhye viśiṣṭāni ṣoḍaśonaṃ śataṃ kṛtam | teṣāṃ madhye

martyaloke dvātriṃśadāsanaṃ śubham || 3

siddhaṃ padmaṃ tathā bhadraṃ muktaṃ vajraṃ ca svastikam |

siṃhaṃ ca gomukhaṃ vīraṃ dhanurāsanameva ca || 4

mṛtaṃ guptaṃ tathā mātsyaṃ matsyendrāsanameva ca | gorakṣaṃ

paścimottānamutkaṭaṃ saṅkaṭaṃ tathā || 5

mayūraṃ kukkuṭaṃ kūrmaṃ tathā cottānakūrmakam |

uttānamaṇḍūkaṃ vṛkṣaṃ maṇḍūkaṃ garuḍaṃ vṛṣam || 6

śalabhaṃ makaraṃ coṣṭraṃ bhujaṅgaṃ ca yogāsanam |

dvātriṃśadāsanāni tu martyaloke hi siddhidam || 7

2.3 -7 The 32 Asanas enumerated for mankind are named:
1_Siddh_asana_verse_2.8 Perfected Pose
2_Padma_asana_verse_2.9 Lotus Pose
3_Bhadra_asana_2.10-11 Strength Pose
4_Mukt_asana_2.12 Liberty Pose

5_Vajra_asana_2.13 Thunderbolt Pose
6_Swastik_asana_2.14 Wellness Pose
https://www.youtube.com/watch?v=YkIAzKczyOk

7_Simh_asana_2.15-16 Lion Pose
8_Gomukh_asana_2.17 Cow's Face Pose
9_Vir_asana_2.18 Brave Pose
10_Dhanur_asana_2.19 Bow Pose
11_Shav_asana_2.20 Relaxation Pose
12_Gupt_asana_2.21 Secrecy Pose
13_Matsy_asana_2.22 Fish Pose
14_(Ardha) Matsyendra_asana_2.23-24 Shark Pose
15_Paschimottan_asana_2.25 Posterior Stretch Pose
16_Goraksh_asana_2.26-27 Shepherd Pose
17_Utkat_asana_2.28 Chair Squat Pose
18_Sankat_asana_2.29 Crisis Pose
https://www.youtube.com/watch?v=QN8GgBfmlmE

19_Mayur_asana_2.30-31 Peacock Pose
20_Kukkut_asana_2.32 Cock Pose
21_Kurma_asana_2.33 Tortoise Pose
22_Uttana_Kurmasana_2.34 Raised Tortoise Pose
23_Manduk_asana_2.35 Frog Pose
24_Uttana_Mandukasana_2.36 Raised Frog Pose
25_Vriksh_asana_2.37 Tree Pose
26_Garud_asana_2.38 Eagle Pose
27_Vrishabh_asana_2.39 Bull Pose
28_Shalabh_asana_2.40 Locust Pose
29_Makar_asana_2 41 Crocodile Pose
30_Ushtr_asana_2.42 Camel Pose
31_Bhujang_asana_2.43-44 Cobra Pose
32_Yog_asana_2.45-46 Yogic Pose

अथ सिद्धासनम् । atha siddhāsanam ।

योनिस्थानकमङ्घ्रिमूलघटितं सम्पीड्य गुल्फेतरं मेढ्रोपर्यथ संनिधाय चिबुकं कृत्वा हृदि
स्थापितम् । स्थाणुः संयमितेन्द्रियोऽचलदृशा पश्यन्भ्रुवोरन्तरे एवं मोक्षविधायते फलकरं
सिद्धासनं प्रोच्यते ॥ ८

2.8 Siddha Asana = Siddhasana = The Perfected Pose
All of us wish to nurture and enhance our talents. The ones who do
exceptionally well become role models in society. Siddhasana
stated here is more than a physical posture. It highlights our innate
desire to become talented, perfected and sought for in our chosen
profession in life.

In this sitting pose one heel is pushing the perineum, and big toe of
other foot is sticking out.

**This pose is specifically for men as it activates the glands for the
male hormones. This is the only pose out of all those mentioned
here that is done with the left leg and right leg in specific
position. We should not alternate the leg position in
Siddhasana. Except for Siddhasana, females can do all the other
asanas in this list.**

Other postures like Ardha Padmasana, Yogasana, Garudasana, etc.
can be done with reversal of legs also.

अथ पद्मासनम् । atha padmāsanam ।
वामोरूपरि दक्षिणं हि चरणं संस्थाप्य वामं तथा दक्षोरूपरि पश्चिमेन विधिना कृत्वा कराभ्यां
दृढम् । अङ्गुष्ठौ हृदये निधाय चिबुकं नासाग्रमालोकये देतद्व्याधिविकारनाशनकरं पद्मासनं
प्रोच्यते ॥ ९
vāmorūpari dakṣiṇam hi caraṇam samsthāpya vāmam tathā

dakṣorūpari paścimena vidhinā kṛtvā karābhyām dṛḍham ।

aṅguṣṭhau hṛdaye nidhāya cibukam nāsāgramālokaye

detadvyādhivikāranāśanakaram padmāsanam procyate ॥ 9
2.9 Padmasana
Apart from being talented, we also wish to be beautiful. The Lotus

flower is coveted for its size, texture, color, beauty and uprightness. In Padmasana we sit cross legged with open feet on our thighs and an erect spine, signifying that one is beautiful from head to toe.

अथ भद्रासनम् । atha bhadrāsanam ।
गुल्फौ च वृषणस्याधो व्युत्क्रमेण समाहितः ।पादाङ्गुष्ठौ कराभ्यां च धृत्वा च पृष्ठदेशतः ॥ १०
जालन्धरं समासाद्य नासाग्रमवलोकयेत् । भद्रासनं भवेदेतत्सर्वव्याधिविनाशकम् ॥ ११
gulphau ca vṛṣaṇasyādho vyutkrameṇa samāhitaḥ ।pādāṅguṣṭhau
karābhyāṃ ca dhṛtvā ca pṛṣṭhadeśataḥ ॥ 10
jālandharaṃ samāsādya nāsāgramavalokayet । bhadrāsanaṃ
bhavedetatsarvavyādhivināśakam ॥ 11
2.10 - 11 Bhadrasana
When one is talented and beautiful, one is empowered to bless the people around us. One innately feels the need to educate and train people and shower grace on mankind.
https://theyogainstitute.org/how-to-do-bhadrasana/

In Bhadrasana, we do a namaste with both feet joined together. It is the pose we all do in butterfly or titliasana.

अथ मुक्तासनम् । atha muktāsanam ।
पायुमूले वामगुल्फं दक्षगुल्फं तथोपरि । समकायशिरोग्रीवं मुक्तासनं तु सिद्धिदम् ॥ १२
pāyumūle vāmagulphaṃ dakṣagulphaṃ tathopari ।
samakāyaśirogrīvaṃ muktāsanaṃ tu siddhidam ॥ 12
2.12 When one has the qualities of skill-beauty and the desire to bless, one achieves liberation from the mundane challenges in day to day life.

In Muktasana we display our freedom from frivolous want, careless craving, and undue negligence.

Muktasana is a composite of Siddhasana and Padmasana, and

much easier to do. It displays the state of liberation one has achieved by practicing the above three asanas.

One heel presses the perineum, the other foot is then comfortably placed on the first thigh.

Liberty is simple and sweet when talent has blossomed, beauty has matured and Grace has showered.

अथ वज्रासनम् । atha vajrāsanam ।

जङ्घाभ्यां वज्रवत्कृत्वा गुदपार्श्वे पदावुभौ । वज्रासनं भवेदेतद्योगिनां सिद्धिदायकम् ॥ १३

jaṅghābhyāṃ vajravatkṛtvā gudapārśve padāvubhau | vajrāsanaṃ

bhavedetadyogināṃ siddhidāyakam ‖ 13

2.13 Vajrasana
When we have everything, when the tummy is full, when the limelight and attention is on us, we need to be humble. One can digest it all, assimilate it properly by sitting in Vajrasana.
A pose of contentment, acceptance, and humility. A pose of surrender to the Lord and Thanksgiving for his grace.

अथ स्वस्तिकासनम् । atha svastikāsanam ।

जानूर्वोरन्तरे कृत्वा योगी पादतले उभे । ऋजुकायः समासीनः स्वस्तिकं तत्प्रचक्षते ॥ १४

jānūrvorantare kṛtvā yogī pādatale ubhe | ṛjukāyaḥ samāsīnaḥ

svastikaṃ tatpracakṣate ‖ 14

2.14 Swastikasana
Wellness beckons and the aura of such a person radiates the inner luminosity.
Common name for this asana is Sukhasana, simple cross-legged sitting posture, which all Indians love to be seated in, and which portrays since ancient times the state of wellness of India.

अथ सिंहासनम् । atha siṃhāsanam ।

गुल्फौ च वृषणस्याधो व्युत्क्रमेणोर्ध्वतां गतौ । चितिमूलौ भूमिसंस्थौ करौ च जानुनोपरि ॥ १५

व्यक्तवक्त्रो जलन्धरं च नासाग्रमवलोकयेत् । सिंहासनं भवेदेतत्सर्वव्याधिविनाशकम् ॥ १६

gulphau ca vṛṣaṇasyādho vyutkrameṇordhvatāṃ gatau | citimūlau

bhūmisaṃsthau karau ca jānunopari || 15

vyaktavaktro jalandharaṃ ca nāsāgramavalokayet | siṃhāsanaṃ

bhavedetatsarvavyādhivināśakam || 16

2.15-16 Simhasana
Now begins the practice of observing peoples and situations
around us, learning how to effectively deal with them.

The Lion has been given the title of king of the forest. And why?
Since its roar travels far and wide, and heralds its arrival to all.
Since its roar comes deep down from the diaphragm and stuns the
opponents.

So we must learn to practice an asana which makes our throat and
voice box strong, which trains our innards to breathe from the
diaphragm.

अथ गोमुखासनम् । atha gomukhāsanam |

पादौ च भूमौ संस्थाप्य पृष्ठपार्श्वे निवेशयेत् । स्थिरकायं समासाद्य गोमुखं गोमुखाऽऽकृतिः ॥ १७

pādau ca bhūmau saṃsthāpya pṛṣṭhapārśve niveśayet | sthirakāyaṃ

samāsādya gomukhaṃ gomukhā"kṛtiḥ || 17

2.17 Gomukhasana = Cow's Face Pose
Along with virtues of a lion, we must nourish the opposite virtues of
innocence and gentleness as a cow.

अथ वीरासनम् । atha vīrāsanam |

एकपादमथैकस्मिन्विन्यसेदूरुसंस्थितम् । इतरस्मिंस्तथा पश्चाद्वीरासनमितीरितम् ॥ १८

ekapādamathaikasminvinyasedūrusaṃsthitam | itarasmiṃstathā

paścādvīrāsanamitīritam || 18
2.18 Virasana = The Brave Pose
Having balanced both the opposing qualities, man becomes
capable of living in this plane of duality, where night and day
coexist, male and female have equal right.

Then alone can a man be said to be brave. And this asana helps
instill bravery and courage in man's heart.

अथ धनुरासनम् | atha dhanurāsanam |
प्रसार्य पादौ भुवि दण्डरूपौ करौ च पृष्ठे धृतपादयुग्मम् ।
कृत्वा धनुस्तुल्यपरिवर्तिताङ्गं निगद्य योगी धनुरासनं तत् ॥ १९
prasārya pādau bhuvi daṇḍarūpau karau ca pṛṣṭhe

dhṛtapādayugmam |

kṛtvā dhanustulyaparivartitāṅgam nigadya yogī dhanurāsanam tat ||
19
2.19 Dhanurasana = Bow Pose
Only a brave man should take up his bow to shoot, since a coward's
aim will always be off target. Dhanurasana helps steady one's hand
when aiming, since it balances the navel and fires up the Manipura
chakra.

अथ शवासनम् | atha śavāsanam |
उत्तानं शववद्भूमौ शयानं तु शवासनम् । शवासनं श्रमहरं चित्तविश्रान्तिकारणम् ॥ २०
uttānam śavavadbhūmau śayānaṃ tu śavāsanam | śavāsanam

śramaharaṃ cittaviśrāntikāraṇam || 20
2.20 Shavasana = Relaxation Pose
After having quelled the opposition, time must be taken for
relaxation, since lots of energy has been expended in the field.
Adrenaline is high, biorhythm is excited, and after being victorious,
one must surely rest to regain inner harmony.

In this pose we release all tenseness, we shut out the external world, we make our breath normal, natural and silent.

अथ गुप्तासनम् । atha guptāsanam ।

जानूर्वोरन्तरे पादौ कृत्वा पादौ च गोपयेत् । पादोपरि च संस्थाप्य गुदं गुप्तासनं विदुः ॥ २१

jānūrvorantare pādau kṛtvā pādau ca gopayet । pādopari ca

saṃsthāpya gudaṃ guptāsanaṃ viduḥ ॥ 21

2.21 Guptasana = Hidden Pose
We release our inhibitors and secrets, by talking to ourselves. This asana makes it easier to bare the soul and stand naked before our own eyes. It thus makes us face ourselves, and that is a great step forward in the world of men.

Sit cross legged, tuck your feet below your bums. You are essentially sitting on the feet and not on the floor.

अथ मत्स्यासनम् । atha matsyāsanam ।

मुक्तपद्मासनं कृत्वा उत्तानशयनं चरेत् । कूर्पराभ्यां शिरो वेष्ट्यं मत्स्यासनं तु रोगहा ॥ २२

muktapadmāsanaṃ kṛtvā uttānaśayanaṃ caret । kūrparābhyāṃ śiro

veṣṭyaṃ matsyāsanaṃ tu rogahā ॥ 22

2.22 Matsyasana = Fish Pose
Fishes are friends with water, such a trait one must also aspire to and attain. Matsyasana helps in making good swimmers, by mimicking a fish and releasing such hormones that aid spending long time in the water or the pool.

अथ मात्स्येन्द्रासनम् । atha mātsyendrāsanam ।

उदरं पश्चिमाभासं कृत्वा तिष्ठति यत्नतः । नम्राङ्गं वामपादं हि दक्षजानूपरि न्यसेत् ॥ २३

तत्र याम्यं कूर्परं च याम्यकरे च वक्रकम् । भ्रुवोर्मध्ये गता दृष्टिः पीठं मात्स्येन्द्रमुच्यते ।

मत्स्येन्द्रपीठं जठराग्निदीप्तं कुर्याद्रोगं च ज्वरा विनाशनम् ॥ २४

udaraṃ paścimābhāsaṃ kṛtvā tiṣṭhati yatnataḥ | namrāṅgaṃ
vāmapādaṃ hi dakṣajānūpari nyaset || 23||
tatra yāmyaṃ kūrparaṃ ca yāmyakare ca vaktrakam |
bhruvormadhye gatā dṛṣṭiḥ pīṭhaṃ mātsyendramucyate |
matsyendrapīṭhaṃ jaṭharāgnidīptaṃ kuryādrogaṃ ca jvarā
vināśanam || 24||
2.23 – 24 Matsyendrasana = Shark Pose = Lord of the Fishes
And in the water if we wish to excel, then Matsyendrasana should
be practiced.

It is good enough to do ardha Matsyendrasana, alternating the leg
and hand positions, so that makes two asanas one after the other.

अथ पश्चिमोत्तानासनम् । atha paścimottānāsanam |
प्रसार्य पादौ भुवि दण्डरूपौ संन्यस्तभालं चितियुग्ममध्ये ।
यत्नेन पादौ च धृतौ कराभ्यां योगीन्द्रपीठं पश्चिमोत्तानमाहुः ॥ २५
prasārya pādau bhuvi daṇḍarūpau saṃnyastabhālaṃ
citiyugmamadhye |
yatnena pādau ca dhṛtau karābhyāṃ yogīndrapīṭhaṃ
paścimottānamāhuḥ || 25
2.25 Paschimottanasan = Posterior Stretch Pose
For many of us the nagging back pain strikes after age 30. This
stretch shall prevent it and also postpone flab from accumulating.

अथ गोरक्षासनम् । atha gorakṣāsanam |
जानूर्वोरन्तरे पादौ उत्तानौ व्यक्तसंस्थितौ ।
गुल्फौ चाच्छाद्य हस्ताभ्यामुत्तानाभ्यां प्रयत्नतः ॥ २६
कण्ठसङ्कोचनं कृत्वा नासाग्रमवलोकयेत् । गोरक्षासनमित्याहुर्योगिनां सिद्धिकारणम् ॥ २७
jānūrvorantare pādau uttānau vyaktasaṃsthitau | gulphau
cācchādya hastābhyāmuttānābhyāṃ prayatnataḥ || 26

kaṇṭhasaṅkocanaṃ kṛtvā nāsāgramavalokayet |

gorakṣāsanamityāhuryogināṃ siddhikāraṇam || 27

2.26 – 27 Gorakshasana = Cowherd or Shepherd Pose
At some time or another we all raise a family, and also need to be a
team leader at work. To strengthen the thoughts and emotions that
shall help in coping up with such pressures, this asana is
recommended.

अथोत्कटासनम् । athotkaṭāsanam |

अङ्गुष्ठाभ्यामवष्टभ्य धरां गुल्फौ च खे गतौ । तत्रोपरि गुदं न्यसेद्विज्ञेयमुत्कटासनम् ॥ २८

aṅguṣṭhābhyāmavaṣṭabhya dharāṃ gulphau ca khe gatau | tatropari

gudaṃ nyasedvijñeyamutkaṭāsanam || 28

2.28 Utkatasana = Chair Squat Pose
Another pose that helps whoever is in charge, whoever is at the
helm, and whoever has to deal with juniors, staff, or raise a family.

The chair pose develops those neural pathways in the brain that
will be needed in decision making affecting many people.

अथ सङ्कटासनम् । atha saṅkaṭāsanam |

वामपादचितेर्मूलं विन्यस्य धरणीतले ।

पाददण्डेन याम्येन वेष्ट्येद्वामपादकम् । जानुयुग्मे करयुग्ममेतत्सङ्कटमासनम् ॥ २९

vāmapādacitermūlaṃ vinyasya dharaṇītale | pādadaṇḍena yāmyena

veṣṭayedvāmapādakam | jānuyugme

karayugmametatsaṅkaṭamāsanam || 29

2.29 Sankatasana = Crisis Pose
A fitting counter pose that supplements and complements the chair
pose. Crisis management, troubleshooting, and fire-fighting
abilities develop with regular practice.

Remember that to achieve any aim the body must be fit and the
mind must be ready. The postures in this set of 32 Asanas are fine-

tuned and especially designed for mankind to develop not only strong muscles and healthy joints, but also nerves of steel.

अथ मयूरासनम् । atha mayūrāsanam ।

धरामवष्टभ्य करयोस्तलाभ्यां तत्कूर्परे स्थापितनाभिपार्श्वम् ।

उच्चासनो दण्डवदुत्थितः खे मयूरमेतत्प्रवदन्ति पीठम् ॥ ३०

बहुकदशनभुक्तं भस्म कुर्यादशेषं जनयति जठराग्निं जारयेत्कालकूटम् ।

हरति सकलरोगानाशु गुल्मज्वरादीन् भवति विगतदोषं ह्यासनं श्रीमयूरम् ॥ ३१

dharāmavaṣṭabhya karayostalābhyāṃ tatkūrpare sthāpitanābhipārśvam ।

uccāsano daṇḍavadutthitaḥ khe mayūrametatpravadanti pīṭham ॥ 30

bahukadaśanabhuktaṃ bhasma kuryādaśeṣaṃ janayati jaṭharāgniṃ jārayetkālakūṭam । harati sakalarogānāśu gulmajvarādīn bhavati vigatadoṣaṃ hyāsanaṃ śrīmayūram ॥ 31

2.30 - 31 Mayurasana = Peacock Pose

Now we see the section of Advanced Asanas. These need to be started at a young age when the muscles and neural pathways are flexible, only then can we perform them once we are past 30 years.

The peacock pose mimics lifting the feet up with hands and face forward like a dancing peacock.

And what are the qualities of a peacock? It eats snakes and scorpions, meaning that it quells poison and vanquishes dangerous foes.

अथ कुक्कुटासनम् । atha kukkuṭāsanam ।

पद्मासनं समासाद्य जानूर्वोरन्तरे करौ । कूर्पराभ्यां समासीनो उच्चस्थः कुक्कुटासनम् ॥ ३२

padmāsanaṃ samāsādya jānūrvorantare karau । kūrparābhyāṃ samāsīno uccasthaḥ kukkuṭāsanam ॥ 32

2.32 Kukkutsana = Rooster Pose
Mimicking a rooster. What does that do? Helps reset the body clock to rise at dawn and go to bed early.

Also imparts virility and handsomeness.

अथ कूर्मासनम् । atha kūrmāsanam ।

गुल्फौ च वृषणस्याधो व्युत्क्रमेण समाहितौ । ऋजुकायशिरोग्रीवं कूर्मासनमितीरितम् ॥ ३३

gulphau ca vṛṣaṇasyādho vyutkrameṇa samāhitau ।

ṛjukāyaśirogrīvaṃ kūrmāsanamitīritam ॥ 33

2.33 Kurmasana = Tortoise Pose

It will enable one to defend well and develop the ability to know when one should recede and fall back instead of continuing to fight. It also allows one to have control over senses, known as dama in Vedanta, one of the six types of wealth.

अथोत्तनकूर्मासनम् । athottanakūrmāsanam ।

कुक्कुटासनबन्धस्थं कराभ्यां धृतकन्धरम् । पीठं कूर्मवदुत्तानमेतदुत्तानकूर्मकम् ॥ ३४

kukkuṭāsanabandhasthaṃ karābhyāṃ dhṛtakandharam । pīṭhaṃ

kūrmavaduttānametaduttānakūrmakam ॥ 34

2.34 Uttana Kurmasana = Raised Tortoise Pose
In knowing when to act and when to stay put, or being intelligent and dumb as the occasion demands, or knowing when to attack and when to surrender, both are needed for raising a happy family or running a large company.

अथ मण्डूकासनम् । atha maṇḍūkāsanam ।

पादतलौ पृष्ठदेशे अङ्गुष्ठे द्वे च संस्पृशेत् । जानुयुग्मं पुरस्कृत्य साधयेन्मण्डूकासनम् ॥ ३५

pādatalau pṛṣṭhadeśe aṅguṣṭhe dve ca saṃspṛśet । jānuyugmaṃ

puraskṛtya sādhayenmaṇḍūkāsanam ॥ 35

2.35 Mandukasana = Frog Pose
Frogs herald rain and abundance, their chatter and jumping about

is clearly evident in the months of July and August. If one can leap with the legs folded, and have such spring in the calf and hip muscles, then know that one can happily enjoy the fruits of one's labor.

अथोत्तनमण्डूकासनम् । athottanamaṇḍūkāsanam ।

मण्डूकासनमध्यस्थं कूर्पराभ्यां धृतं शिरः । एतद्भेकवदुत्तानमेतदुत्तानमण्डूकम् ॥ ३६

maṇḍūkāsanamadhyasthaṃ kūrparābhyāṃ dhṛtaṃ śiraḥ ।

etadbhekavaduttānametaduttānamaṇḍūkam ॥ 36

2.36 Uttana Mandukasana = Raised Frog Pose
A variation that is an advanced posture, and that signifies that one is going to reap the fruits of labor even after having advanced in age. Normally the time when one should be happily at home one is seen to spend in nursing care or as an invalid, with no chance of any enjoyment nor relaxation. This advanced posture if once can begin at a young age, then old age is destined to be relaxed.

अथ वृक्षासनम् । atha vṛkṣāsanam ।

वामोरुमूलदेशे च याम्यं पादं निधाय तु । तिष्ठेत्तु वृक्षवद्भूमौ वृक्षासनमिदं विदुः ॥ ३७

vāmorumūladeśe ca yāmyaṃ pādaṃ nidhāya tu । tiṣṭhettu

vṛkṣavadbhūmau vṛkṣāsanamidaṃ viduḥ ॥ 37

2.37 Vrikshasana = Tree Pose
Tree has many nerves and veins that supply sap to all its branches and leaves, hence flowers sprout and fruits are laden. This pose has been designed to give ample reflex and massage to all tubes in the body, such that the farthest limbs, (fingers and toes and hair), all remain functional, lustrous and healthy.

अथ गरुडासनम् । atha garuḍāsanam ।

जङ्घोरुभ्यां धरां पीड्य स्थिरकायो द्विजानुना । जानूपरि करयुग्मं गरुडासनमुच्यते ॥ ३८

jaṅghorubhyāṃ dharāṃ pīḍya sthirakāyo dvijānunā । jānūpari

karayugmaṃ garuḍāsanamucyate ॥ 38

2.38 Garudasana = Eagle Pose

An eagle soars the highest, and has a long-range vision too. This asana can help visionaries and leaders develop the necessary qualities to govern from the helm and perform their tasks with foresight and be aware of what is happening in their lowest ranks and file. It will also ensure availability of vehicles for speedy travel to long distances.

अथ वृषासनम् । atha vṛṣāsanam / vrishabhasana

याम्यगुल्फे पायुमूलं वामभागे पदेतरम् । विपरीतं स्पृशेद्धूर्मि वृषासनमिदं भवेत् ॥ ३९

yāmyagulphe pāyumūlaṃ vāmabhāge padetaram | viparītaṃ

spṛśedbhūmiṃ vṛṣāsanamidaṃ bhavet ‖ 39

2.39 Vrishabhasana = Bull Pose

Grand, complex, and high aim designs are never achieved without dogged struggle, and they also take sufficient length of time for successful completion. A bull has the qualities of working day in and day out, without slackening strength or tempo.
https://www.tummee.com/yoga-poses/vrishabhasana
The Vrishabhasana can be done by anyone since it is a beginner level posture, yet it has the most remarkable effect on the entire lower body from waist downwards. These are the organs and limbs needed for continuous sitting, cycling, walking, or labor, and also for digestion and excretion. Even expectant mothers can benefit a lot from this asana.

अथ शलभासनम् । atha śalabhāsanam |

अध्यास्य शेते करयुग्मं वक्षे भूमिमवष्टभ्य करयोस्तलाभ्याम् ।

पादौ च शून्ये च वितस्ति चोर्ध्वं वदन्ति पीठं शलभं मुनीन्द्राः ॥ ४०

adhyāsya śete karayugmaṃ vakṣe bhūmimavaṣṭabhya

karayostalābhyām |

pādau ca śūnye ca vitasti cordhvaṃ vadanti pīṭhaṃ śalabhaṃ

munīndrāḥ ‖ 40

2.40 Shalabhasana = Locust Pose

Another simple yet amazingly effective asana is the Shalabhasana. All of us from young children to hectic businessmen to wizened grandmothers can do it. And it imparts long term flexibility and postural correctness to the organs and joints below the waist. Locusts never age. They fly and hop with the same alacrity till the end. We must all learn and do this asana daily. Remember to stretch your lifted leg(s) in the direction of the feet, as if someone is pulling your leg! When we ourselves become good at physical leg-pulling, no amount of outside disturbances can throw us off balance.

अथ मकरासनम् । atha makarāsanam ।

अध्यास्य शेते हृदयं निधाय भूमौ च पादौ च प्रसार्यमाणौ ।

शिरश्च धृत्वा करदण्डयुग्मे देहाग्निकारं मकरासनं तत् ॥ ४१

adhyāsya śete hṛdayaṃ nidhāya bhūmau ca pādau ca prasāryamāṇau ।

śiraśca dhṛtvā karadaṇḍayugme dehāgnikāraṃ makarāsanaṃ tat ॥ 41

2.41 Makarasana = Crocodile Pose

This is the asana to raise the ojas in our being, and feel tough and full inside. Crocodiles are prehistoric mammals from long ago, that learnt to live deep inside the waters, on the surface of the waters, and on land. Their resilience to nature's storms and spoils is legendary, and they can be found both in fresh water lakes and rivers, and in the salty oceans. Makarasana lends a quality of indestructibility to the being, and is so simple that none can claim they cannot do it.

In fact most of us are curled up in makarasana while lying down on our belly. It is a de facto favorite of teens, youngsters, or babies. Better to keep on doing it past one's prime.

अथोष्ट्रासनम् । athoṣṭrāsanam ।

अध्यास्य शेते पदयुग्ममव्यस्तं पृष्ठे निधायापि धृतं कराभ्याम् ।

आकुञ्चयेत्सम्यगुदरास्यगाढमौष्ट्रं च पीठं योगिनो वदन्ति ॥ ४२

adhyāsya śete padayugmavyastaṃ pṛṣṭhe nidhāyāpi dhṛtaṃ karābhyām |

ākuñcayetsamyagudarāsyagāḍhamauṣṭraṃ ca pīṭhaṃ yogino vadanti ॥ 42

2.42 Ushtrasana = Camel Pose

Difficulty, Hunger, Starvation, the camel takes it all in its stride. How? Because it prepares well when things are easy and plentiful. Doing ushtrasana regularly will keep any and all illnesses at bay, and help the body cope up with missing meals if the situation so arises. This is an advanced asana, and needs proper training and guidance initially.

अथ भुजङ्गासनम् । atha bhujaṅgāsanam |

अङ्गुष्ठनाभिपर्यन्तमधोभूमौ विनिन्यसेत् । करतलाभ्यां धरां धृत्वोर्ध्वं शीर्षं फणीव हि ॥ ४३
देहाग्निर्वर्धते नित्यं सर्वरोगविनाशनम् । जागर्ति भुजगी देवी साधनाद्भुजङ्गासनम् ॥ ४४ ॥

aṅgusthanābhiparyantamadhobhūmau vininyaset | karatalābhyāṃ dharāṃ dhṛtvordhvaṃ śīrṣaṃ phaṇīva hi ॥ 43

dehāgnirvardhate nityaṃ sarvarogavināśanam | jāgarti bhujagī devī sādhanādbhujaṅgāsanam ॥ 44

2.43 – 44 Bhujangasana = Cobra Pose

If one can asks TELL ME ONLY ONE ASANA that is absolutely a must for reliability of physical and mental fitness in the long run, then Bhujang Asana takes the pride of place. It is the King of all Asanas. It has been taught in ashrams, gurukuls and traditional Vedanta centers since the very beginning, and all of us are encouraged to start doing the Cobra Pose for developing a sharp intellect, guts in the heart, and digestive fire.

Notice that even this asana is simpler and readily doable for all members of the family. Notice the Vision of Rishi Gheranda, who successively places the simpler Asanas towards the end, and the best asana is at the very end.

Why? When one is young, one may be able to do all these 32 asanas properly. However as one touches middle age, only around 12 asanas of these 32 can be done gracefully, and they are good enough if the growing up years have been a bit disciplined.

The 12 asanas for every age group are:
i) 4_Mukt_asana_2.12 Liberty Pose
ii) 5_Vajra_asana_2.13 Thunderbolt Pose
iii) 6_Swastik_asana_2.14 Wellness Pose
iv) 7_Simh_asana_2.15-16 Lion Pose
v) 9_Vir_asana_2.18 Brave Pose
vi) 11_Shav_asana_2.20 Relaxation Pose
vii) 25_Vrikshasana_2.37 Tree Pose
viii) 27_Vrishabasana_2.39 Bull Pose
ix) 28_Shalabhasana_2.40 Locust Pose
x) 29_Makarasana_2 41 Crocodile Pose
xi) 31_Bhujangasana_2.43-44 Cobra Pose
xii) 32_Yogasana_2.45-46 Yogic Pose
 (for some of us one or two asanas can be interchanged in this set)

अथ योगासनम् । atha yogāsanam ।

उत्तानौ चरणौ कृत्वा संस्थाप्य जानुनोपरि।आसनोपरि संस्थाप्य चोत्तानं करयुग्मकम्॥४५

पूरकैर्वायुमाकृष्य नासाग्रमवलोकयेत् । योगासनं भवेदेतद्योगिनां योगसाधने ॥ ४६

uttānau caraṇau kṛtvā saṃsthāpya jānunopari।āsanopari saṃsthāpya

cottānaṃ karayugmakam ॥ 45

pūrakairvāyumākṛṣya nāsāgramavalokayet । yogāsanaṃ

bhavedetadyogināṃ yogasādhane ॥ 46

2.45 – 46 Yogasana = Yogic Pose
We have noticed that the famous temples have shown the idols of Shiva, Buddha or a Saint with eyes half closed and the gaze directed at 30 degrees towards the floor. (i.e. towards the tip of the nose). When one becomes an advanced Meditator, and starts to reap its rich benefits, one finds that automatically one's gaze drops

down, and one's eyes droop.

Such a comfortable sitting posture with open palms facing the sky and gaze directed at 30 degrees is called the Yogic Pose, since it is natural with saints and seers, who are no longer entangled with this visible creation, and hence are not hampered by it in any way. It does not mean that we stop any activity. On the other hand, we pursue all our duties and responsibilities with gusto and live a highly creative, productive and fulfilling life, but we know at the back of the mind that it is all a temporary dream. So, it keeps our mind safe and shielded from the storms and upheavals and un-pleasantries. It keeps us distanced from bitterness and frustration. It keeps us free of dangerous notions that someone is bad or corrupt or harmful, when we fail to appreciate the fundamental law of nature - OPPOSITE VALUES ARE COMPLEMENTARY IN CREATION.

॥ इति श्री घेरण्डसंहितायां महर्षि-घेरण्ड-नृप-चण्डकापालि-संवादे घटस्थयोगे द्वात्रिंशासनवर्णनं नाम द्वितीयोपदेशः ॥ iti śrī gheraṇḍasaṃhitāyāṃ maharṣi-gheraṇḍa-nṛpa-caṇḍakāpāli-saṃvāde ghaṭasthayoge dvātriṃśāsanavarṇanaṃ nāma dvitīyopadeśaḥ ॥

Here ends the 2nd chapter of the dialogue named Gheranda Samhita, the teaching of Maharshi Gheranda to king Chandakapali.

3 Gestures - Mudra मुद्राप्रयोगो नाम तृतीयोपदेशः

घेरण्ड उवाच । gheraṇḍa uvāca ।

महामुद्रा नभोमुद्रा उड्डीयानं जलन्धरम् । मूलबन्धं महाबन्धं महावेधश्च खेचरी ॥ १

विपरीतकरी योनिर्वज्रोली शक्तिचालनी । ताडागी माण्डुकीमुद्रा शाम्भवी पञ्चधारणा ॥ २

अश्विनी पाशिनी काकी मातङ्गी च भुजङ्गिनी । पञ्चविंशतिमुद्राश्च सिद्धिदा इह योगिनाम् ॥३

mahāmudrā nabhomudrā uḍḍīyānaṃ jalandharam | mūlabandhaṃ

mahābandhaṃ mahāvedhaśca khecarī ‖ 1

viparītakarī yonirvajrolī śakticālanī | tāḍāgī māṇḍukīmudrā śāmbhavī

pañcadhāraṇā ‖ 2

aśvinī pāśinī kākī mātaṅgī ca bhujaṅginī | pañcaviṃśatimudrāśca

siddhidā iha yoginām ‖ 3

3.1-3 There are 25 Mudras and Bandhas and Dharanas.

- Mudra is a gesture using our hands and fingers.
- Bandha is a lock, by contracting specific muscles we seal the body exits.
- Dharana is a mental Imagination that we use to focus our thoughts.

All these three we must learn for proper functioning of our Chakras. These serve to channelize the prana and consciousness through certain pathways by making circuits within the body. These circuits are powerful mechanisms for quickly increasing the energy and vitality. In turn many illnesses get subdued, cured or prevented.

These are named
1_Maha Mudra_3.6,7,8
2_Nabho Mudra_3.9
3_Uddiyana Bandha_3.10, 11
4_Jalandhar Bandha_3.12, 13
5_Moola Bandha_3.14, 15, 16, 17
6_Maha Bandha_3.18, 19, 20
7_Maha Vedha_3.21, 22, 23, 24

अथ मुद्राणां फलकथनम् । atha mudrāṇām phalakathanam ।

मुद्राणां पटलं देवि कथितं तव संनिधौ । येन विज्ञातमात्रेण सर्वसिद्धिः प्रजायते ॥ ४

गोपनीयं प्रयत्नेन न देयं यस्य कस्यचित् । प्रीतिदं योगिनां चैव दुर्लभं मरुतामपि ॥ ५

mudrāṇāṃ paṭalaṃ devi kathitaṃ tava saṃnidhau । yena

vijñātamātreṇa sarvasiddhiḥ prajāyate ॥ 4

gopanīyaṃ prayatnena na deyaṃ yasya kasyacit । prītidaṃ yogināṃ

caiva durlabhaṃ marutāmapi ॥ 5

3.4-5 I have overhead a chat between Auspiciousness and Beauty.
Auspicious remarked, your beauty has grown a thousand-fold since
you started Mudra practice. And I am sure your talents have
multiplied as well.
And Beauty replied, certainly this is most remarkable I have
noticed, and it has taken lots of sustained effort, adherence to
discipline and timing, and patient practice over an entire year to
achieve.
Even the seasons around me have become favorable as a result.

अथ महामुद्राकथनम् । atha mahāmudrākathanam ।

पायुमूलं वामगुल्फे संपीड्य दृढयत्नतः । याम्यपादं प्रसार्याथ करे धृतपदाङ्गुलः ॥ ६

कण्ठसङ्कोचनं कृत्वा भ्रुवोर्मध्यं निरीक्षयेत् । महामुद्राभिधा मुद्रा कथ्यते चैव सूरिभिः ॥ ७

अथ महामुद्राफलकथनम् । atha mahāmudrāphalakathanam ।

वलितं पलितं चैव जरां मृत्युं निवारयेत् । क्षयकासं गुदावर्तं प्लीहाजीर्णं ज्वरं तथा ।

नाशयेत्सर्वरोगांश्च महामुद्रा च साधनात् ॥ ८

pāyumūlaṃ vāmagulphe saṃpīḍya dṛḍhayatnataḥ | yāmyapādaṃ

prasāryātha kare dhṛtapadāṅgulaḥ ‖ 6

kaṇṭhasaṅkocanaṃ kṛtvā bhruvormadhyaṃ nirīkṣayet |

mahāmudrābhidhā mudrā kathyate caiva sūribhiḥ ‖ 7

atha mahāmudrāphalakathanam | valitaṃ palitaṃ caiva jarāṃ

mṛtyuṃ nivārayet | kṣayakāsaṃ gudāvartaṃ plīhājīrṇaṃ jvaraṃ

tathā | nāśayetsarvarogāṃśca mahāmudrā ca sādhanāt ‖ 8

3.6-8 Make sure you sit in a manner that is comfortable and suitable. Then direct your gaze towards your open palms. Sit long enough so that the breath becomes silent, the gaze becomes unwavering, and the posture remains immobile.

Such practice of Mahamudra surely prohibits temptation, bowel movement is restored, the activity of the spleen is strengthened, and unfavorable thoughts from the mind are banished.

Overall health gets quickly restored.

अथ नभोमुद्राकथनम् । atha nabhomudrākathanam ।

यत्र यत्र स्थितो योगी सर्वकार्येषु सर्वदा । ऊर्ध्वजिह्वः स्थिरो भूत्वा धारयेत्पवनं सदा ।

नभोमुद्रा भवेदेषा योगिनां रोगनाशिनी ॥ ९

yatra yatra sthito yogī sarvakāryeṣu sarvadā | ūrdhvajihvaḥ sthiro

bhūtvā dhārayetpavanaṃ sadā | nabhomudrā bhavedeṣā yogināṃ

roganāśinī ‖ 9

3.9 Curling the tongue up and back to touch the soft palate, and making the breath smooth, and doing likewise many times in a day, triggers the cure of certain illnesses.

This is named Nabho Mudra for the Nabhi or Navel Hub.

अथ उड्डीयानकथनम् । atha uḍḍīyānakathanam ।

उदरे पश्चिमं तानं नाभेरूर्ध्वं तु कारयेत् । उड्डीनं कुरुते यस्मादविश्रान्तं महाखगः ।
उड्डीयानं त्वसौ बन्धो मृत्युमातङ्गकेसरी ॥ १०

अथोड्डीयानबन्धस्य फलकथनम् । समग्राद्बन्धनाच्येतदुड्डीयानं विशिष्यते ।
उड्डीयाने समभ्यस्ते मुक्तिः स्वाभाविकी भवेत् ॥ ११

udare paścimaṃ tānaṃ nābherūrdhvaṃ tu kārayet । uḍḍīnaṃ

kurute yasmādaviśrāntaṃ mahākhagaḥ । uḍḍīyānaṃ tvasau bandho

mṛtyumātaṅgakesarī ॥ 10

athoḍḍīyānabandhasya phalakathanam ।

samagrādbandhanāddhyetaduḍḍīyānaṃ viśiṣyate । uḍḍīyāne

samabhyaste muktiḥ svābhāvikī bhavet ॥ 11

3.10-11 Uddiyan Bandh is done by raising the stomach muscles up
and pulling them back.
It's sustained practice will keep ageing at bay, and make the body
feel light as a bird.
Uddiyana Bandha is especially useful for all age groups.

अथ जालन्धरबन्धकथनम् । atha jālandharabandhakathanam ।

कण्ठसङ्कोचनं कृत्वा चिबुकं हृदये न्यसेत् । जालन्धरे कृते बन्धे षोडशाधारबन्धनम् ।
जालन्धरमहामुद्रा मृत्योश्च क्षयकारिणी ॥ १२

अथ जालन्धरबन्धस्य फलकथनम् । सिद्धे जालन्धरे बन्धे योगिनां सिद्धिदायकम् ।
षण्मासमभ्यसेद्यो हि स सिद्धो नाऽत्र संशयः ॥ १३

kaṇṭhasaṅkocanaṃ kṛtvā cibukaṃ hṛdaye nyaset । jālandhare kṛte

bandhe ṣoḍaśādhārabandhanam । jālandharamahāmudrā mṛtyośca

kṣayakāriṇī ॥ 12

atha jālandharabandhasya phalakathanam । siddhaṃ jālandharaṃ bandhaṃ yogināṃ siddhidāyakam | ṣaṇmāsamabhyasedyo hi sa

siddho nā'tra saṃśayaḥ ‖ 13

3.12-13 Engaging the throat muscles, bring the chin to the chest.
This is known as Jalandhar Bandha; it prevents the sixteen types of
faulty speech.

When Jalandhar Bandha is applied with Maha Mudra, the ageing is
delayed.

It takes six months to become adept in applying the Jalandhar
Bandha. Success is then rapidly ensured as the tongue gets
tempered.

अथ मूलबन्धकथनम् | atha mūlabandhakathanam |

पार्ष्णिना वामपादस्य योनिमाकुञ्चयेत्ततः। नाभिग्रन्थि मेरुदण्डे संपीड्य यत्नतः सुधीः ॥१४

मेढ्रं दक्षिणगुल्फे तु दृढबन्धं समाचरेत् । नाभेरूर्ध्वमधश्चापि तानं कुर्यात्प्रयत्नतः ।

जराविनाशिनी मुद्रा मूलबन्धो निगद्यते ॥ १५

pārṣṇinā vāmapādasya yonimākuñcayettataḥ | nābhigranthiṃ

merudaṇḍe saṃpīḍya yatnataḥ sudhīḥ ‖ 14

meḍhraṃ dakṣiṇagulphe tu dṛḍhabandhaṃ samācaret |

nābherūrdhvamadhaścāpi tānaṃ kuryātprayatnataḥ | jarāvināśinī

mudrā mūlabandho nigadyate ‖ 15

3.14-15 Expelling the air from the abdomen and intestines, contract
the anal muscles as if preventing and delaying the discharge.

This is known as Moola Bandha, and it ensures good health even in
old age.

अथ मूलबन्धस्य फलकथनम् | atha mūlabandhasya phalakathanam |

संसारसमुद्रं तर्तुमभिलषति यः पुमान् । विरले सुगुप्तो भूत्वा मुद्रामेतां समभ्यसेत् ॥ १६

अभ्यासाद्बन्धनस्यास्य मरुत्सिद्धिर्भवेद्ध्रुवम्।साधयेच्चलतस्तर्हि मौनी तु विजिताऽलसः ॥ १७

saṃsārasamudraṃ tartumabhilaṣati yaḥ pumān | virale sugupto
bhūtvā mudrāmetāṃ samabhyaset || 16
abhyāsādbandhanasyāsya marutsiddhirbhaveddhruvam |
sādhayedyatnatastarhi maunī tu vijitā'lasaḥ || 17
3.16-17 It is best to apply the above three bandhas in sequence,
beginning with Mooladhar, then Uddiyan and finally Jalandhar.

Hold the Jalandhar for least time, and Mooladhar for the maximum
time.

Ensure diligence, silence and limited contact while doing these
practices, since that will help in greater control over the breath and
thus ensure success.

अथ महाबन्धकथनम् । atha mahābandhakathanam |
वामपादस्य गुल्फेन पायुमूलं निरोधयेत् । दक्षपादेन तद्गुल्फं संपीड्य यत्नतः सुधीः ॥ १८
शनैः शनैश्चालयेत्पार्ष्णिं योनिमाकुञ्चयेच्छनैः । जालन्धरे धारयेत्प्राणं महाबन्धो निगद्यते
॥ १९

अथ महाबन्धस्य फलकथनम् । atha mahābandhasya phalakathanam |
महाबन्धः परो बन्धो जरामरणनाशनः । प्रसादादस्य बन्धस्य साधयेत्सर्ववाञ्छितम् ॥ २०
vāmapādasya gulphena pāyumūlaṃ nirodhayet | dakṣapādena
tadgulphaṃ saṃpīḍya yatnataḥ sudhīḥ || 18
śanaiḥ śanaiścālayetpārṣṇiṃ yonimākuñcayecchanaiḥ | jālandhare
dhārayetprāṇaṃ mahābandho nigadyate || 19
mahābandhaḥ paro bandho jarāmaraṇanāśanaḥ | prasādādasya
bandhasya sādhayetsarvavāñcitam || 20
3.18-20 Mahabandh is the sequential and simultaneous application
of Moolbandh, Uddiyanbandh and Jalandhar bandh, and then the
sequential release of Jalandhar, Uddiyana, and Moolbandh
respectively.

Mahabandh is highly recommended to extricate oneself from inactivity, suffering or depression. That in turn gives positive direction to life and ensures success in all ventures.

अथ महावेधकथनम् । atha mahāvedhakathanam ।
रूपयौवनलावण्यं नारीणां पुरुषं विना । मूलबन्धमहाबन्धौ महावेधं विना तथा ॥ २१
महाबन्धं समासाद्य उड्डानकुम्भकं चरेत् ।महावेधः समाख्यातो योगिनां सिद्धिदायकः ॥२२
अथ महावेधस्य फलकथनम् । atha mahāvedhasya phalakathanam ।
महाबन्धमूलबन्धौ महावेधसमन्वितौ । प्रत्यहं कुरुते यस्तु स योगी योगवित्तमः ॥ २३
न मृत्युतो भयं तस्य न जरा तस्य विद्यते । गोपनीयः प्रयत्नेन वेधोऽयं योगिपुङ्गवैः ॥ २४
rūpayauvanalāvaṇyam nārīṇāṃ puruṣaṃ vinā |

mūlabandhamahābandhau mahāvedhaṃ vinā tathā ‖ 21

mahābandhaṃ samāsādya uḍḍānakumbhakaṃ caret |mahāvedhaḥ

samākhyāto yoginām siddhidāyakaḥ ‖ 22

atha mahāvedhasya phalakathanam | mahābandhamūlabandhau

mahāvedhasamanvitau | pratyaham kurute yastu sa yogī

yogavittamaḥ ‖ 23

na mṛtyuto bhayaṃ tasya na jarā tasya vidyate | gopanīyaḥ

prayatnena vedho'yaṃ yogipuṅgavaiḥ ‖ 24

3.21-24 Mahabandh is really effective when done with the air expelled from the stomach and then holding the breath as long as comfortable.

Remember that Mahabandh will also enhance the charms of a woman, and make her more alluring to men and vice versa.

This is known as Maha Vedha, it ensures a successful marriage, and getting along of couples.

Perfect Union is the result, harmony and cooperation is easily achieved. Thoughts of separation or loss are vanquished.

जिह्वाऽधो नाडीं सच्छिन्नां रसनां चालयेत्सदा । दोहयेन्नवनीतेन लौहयन्त्रेण कर्षयेत् ॥ २५

एवं नित्यं समभ्यासाल्लम्बिका दीर्घतां व्रजेत्।यावद्गच्छेद्भ्रुवोर्मध्ये तदा गच्छति खेचरी॥२६

रसनां तालुमध्ये तु शनैः शनैः प्रवेशयेत् । कपालकुहरे जिह्वा प्रविष्टा विपरीतगा ।

भ्रुवोर्मध्ये गता दृष्टिमुद्रा भवति खेचरी ॥ २७

अथ खेचरी मुद्रायाः फलकथनम् । न च मूर्च्छा क्षुधा तृष्णा नैवाऽऽलस्यं प्रजायते ।

न च रोगो जरा मृत्युर्देवदेहः स जायते ॥ २८

न चाग्निर्दहते गात्रं न शोषयति मारुतः । न देहं क्लेदयन्त्यापो दंशयेन्न भुजङ्गमः ॥ २९

लावण्यं च भवेद्गात्रे समाधिर्जायते ध्रुवम् । कपालवक्रसंयोगे रसना रसमाप्नुयात् ॥ ३०

नानारससमुद्भूतमानन्दं च दिने दिने । आदौ लवणक्षारं च ततस्तिक्तकषायकम् ॥ ३१

jihvā'dho nāḍīṃ sañcinnāṃ rasanāṃ cālayetsadā |

dohayennavanītena lauhayantreṇa karṣayet || 25

evaṃ nityaṃ samabhyāsāllambikā dīrghatāṃ vrajet |

yāvadgacchedbhruvormadhye tadā gacchati khecarī || 26

rasanāṃ tālumadhye tu śanaiḥ śanaiḥ praveśayet | kapālakuhare

jihvā praviṣṭā viparītagā | bhruvormadhye gatā dṛṣṭirmudrā bhavati

khecarī || 27

atha khecarī mudrāyāḥ phalakathanam | na ca mūrcchā kṣudhā

tṛṣṇā naivā"lasyaṃ prajāyate | na ca rogo jarā mṛtyurdevadehaḥ sa

jāyate || 28

na cāgnirdahate gātraṃ na śoṣayati mārutaḥ | na dehaṃ

kledayantyāpo daṃśayenna bhujaṅgamaḥ || 29

lāvaṇyaṃ ca bhavedgātre samādhirjāyate dhruvam |

kapālavaktrasaṃyoge rasanā rasamāpnuyāt || 30

nānārasasamudbhūtamānandaṃ ca dine dine | ādau lavaṇakṣāraṃ

ca tatastiktakaṣāyakam || 31

3.25-31 Kechhari Mudra is done by elongating the tongue and
rubbing it lightly on a point in the soft palate.
This is the point where the tendon is clearly felt beneath the soft

flesh. It is point of union of the five tastes.

नवनीतं घृतं क्षीरं दधितक्रमधूनि च । द्राक्षारसं च पीयूषं जायते रसनोदकम् ॥ ३२

navanītaṃ ghṛtaṃ kṣīraṃ dadhitakramadhūni ca | drākṣārasaṃ ca

pīyūṣaṃ jāyate rasanodakam || 32

3.32 Salty, bitter, bland are the tastes that initially occupy our attention since they represent the basic needs and emotions. Once satisfied, one moves to experience the primordial tastes of butter, ghee, milk, curd and buttermilk as had by us in our babyhood. These regenerate the sensations of sweet trust, and finally the bliss of divine nectar is experienced.

अथ विपरीतकरणीमुद्राकथनम् । atha viparītakaraṇīmudrākathanam |

नाभिमूले वसेत्सूर्यस्तालुमूले च चन्द्रमाः । अमृतं ग्रसते सूर्यस्ततो मृत्युवशो नरः ॥ ३३

ऊर्ध्वं च योजयेत्सूर्यं चन्द्रं च अध आनयेत् । विपरीतकरी मुद्रा सर्वतन्त्रेषु गोपिता ॥ ३४

भूमौ शिरश्च संस्थाप्य करयुग्मं समाहितः । ऊर्ध्वपादः स्थिरो भूत्वा विपरीतकरी मता ॥ ३५

nābhimūle vasetsūryastālumūle ca candramāḥ | amṛtaṃ grasate

sūryastato mṛtyuvaśo naraḥ || 33

ūrdhvaṃ ca yojayetsūryaṃ candraṃ ca adha ānayet | viparītakarī

mudrā sarvatantreṣu gopitā || 34

bhūmau śiraśca saṃsthāpya karayugmaṃ samāhitaḥ | ūrdhvapādaḥ

sthiro bhūtvā viparītakarī matā || 35

3.33-35 Viparit Karani is an upward tilt of the legs to 135 degrees, hands supported on the bums.

We associate heat with the navel pit that separates the diaphragm breath from the stomach food, and cold with our palate that separates the nasal cavity from the mouth.

Generally the cold is above in the cerebellum and the heat is below in the stomach pit, so viparit karani is the easiest asana to reverse the two and thereby balance them for people of all age groups.

अथ विपरीतकरणीमुद्रायाः फलकथनम् । atha viparītakaraṇīmudrāyāḥ phalakathanam ।

मुद्रां च साधयेन्नित्यं जरां मृत्युं च नाशयेत्। स सिद्धः सर्वलोकेषु प्रलयेऽपि न सीदति ॥३६

mudrāṃ ca sādhayennityaṃ jarāṃ mṛtyuṃ ca nāśayet । sa siddhaḥ sarvalokeṣu pralaye'pi na sīdati ॥ 36

3.36 Most asanas of real benefit have to be learnt and practiced at a young age. However, Viparit Karani has been mentioned in this section since even though it's an Asana, it can be done at any age and in any physical state.

अथ योनिमुद्राकथनम् । atha yonimudrākathanam ।

सिद्धासनं समासाद्य कर्णाक्षिनासिकामुखम् । अङ्गुष्ठतर्जनीमध्यानामादिभिश्च धारयेत् ॥३७

काकीभिः प्राणं सङ्कृष्य अपाने योजयेत्ततः । षट्चक्राणि क्रमाद्ध्यात्वा हुं हंसमनुना सुधीः॥३८

चैतन्यमानयेद्देवीं निद्रिता या भुजङ्गिनी । जीवेन सहितां शक्तिं समुत्थाप्य पराम्बुजे ॥ ३९

शक्तिमयः स्वयं भूत्वा परं शिवेन सङ्गमम् । नानासुखं विहारं च चिन्तयेत्परमं सुखम् ॥४०

शिवशक्तिसमायोगादेकान्तं भुवि भावयेत्।आनन्दमानसो भूत्वा अहं ब्रह्मेति सम्भवेत्॥४१

योनिमुद्रा परा गोप्या देवानामपि दुर्लभा । सकृत्तु लाभसंसिद्धिः समाधिस्थः स एव हि॥४२

siddhāsanaṃ samāsādya karṇākṣināsikāmukham ।

aṅguṣṭhatarjanīmadhyānāmādibhiśca dhārayet ॥ 37

kākībhiḥ prāṇaṃ saṅkṛṣya apāne yojayettataḥ । ṣaṭcakraṇi kramāddhyātvā huṃ haṃsamanunā sudhīḥ ॥ 38

caitanyamānayeddevīṃ nidritā yā bhujaṅginī । jīvena sahitāṃ śaktiṃ samutthāpya parāmbuje ॥ 39

śaktimayaḥ svayaṃ bhūtvā paraṃ śivena saṅgamam । nānāsukhaṃ vihāraṃ ca cintayetparamaṃ sukham ॥ 40

śivaśaktisamāyogādekāntaṃ bhuvi bhāvayet।ānandamānaso bhūtvā ahaṃ brahmeti sambhavet ॥ 41

yonimudrā parā gopyā devānāmapi durlabhā | sakṛttu
lābhasaṃsiddhiḥ samādhisthaḥ sa eva hi || 42
3.37-42 Be seated in a posture that is immobile as well as
comfortable. Legs firmly grounded, spine straight.

Now apply Shanmukhi Mudra, thumbs at ears, index finger on
eyebrows, middle finger at nostrils, ring finger on upper lips, little
finger near chin.

Breathe in silently through the nose, press all the marma points
with the finger tips, then make the "hum" ह्रूँ humming bee sound
while releasing the breath.

Do it for three to six breaths, enjoying the cooling reverberations at
the back of the head. Know that all senses get satiated with this
practice, and the relaxation obtained ensures sound sleep.

This Shanmukhi Mudra can be done sitting, lying down, standing or
walking and hence gets the name Yoni Mudra, or the Mudra that
delivers pleasurable sensations akin to romantic touch.

These experiences are of the subtle and can be confused with
deeper states.

अथ योनिमुद्राफलकथनम् | atha yonimudrāphalakathanam |
ब्रह्महा भ्रूणहा चैव सुरापी गुरुतल्पगः । एतैः पापैर्न लिप्येत योनिमुद्रानिबन्धनात् || ४३
यानि पापानि घोराणि उपपापानि यानि च । तानि सर्वाणि नश्यन्ति योनिमुद्रानिबन्धनात् ।
तस्मादभ्यसनं कुर्याद्यदि मुक्तिं समिच्छति || ४४

brahmahā bhrūṇahā caiva surāpī gurutalpagaḥ | etaiḥ pāpairna
lipyeta yonimudrānibandhanāt || 43
yāni pāpāni ghorāṇi upapāpāni yāni ca | tāni sarvāṇi naśyanti
yonimudrānibandhanāt | tasmādabhyasanaṃ kuryādyadi muktiṃ
samicchati || 44

3.43-44 One may escape the conjugal temptations of sleeping with the neighbor's wife, and avoid serious lustful desires by a proper and sustained practice of the Yoni Mudra. One can get the excitement of romance, of roaming distant lands, of having dangerous adventures, and thus satisfy one's craving without incurring the associated guilt and physical downfall.

अथ वज्रोलिमुद्राकथनम् । atha vajrolimudrākathanam ।
धरामवष्टभ्य करयोस्तलाभ्या मूर्ध्वं क्षिपेत्पादयुगं शिरः खे ।
शक्तिप्रबोधाय चिरजीवनाय वज्रोलिमुद्रां मुनयो वदन्ति ॥ ४५
dharāmavaṣṭabhya karayostalābhyā mūrdhvaṃ kṣipetpādayugaṃ

śiraḥ khe । śaktiprabodhāya cirajīvanāya vajrolimudrāṃ munayo

vadanti ॥ 45

3.45 Sit straight with palms firmly planted on the ground, feet together and legs straight. Now lift up both the legs in the air, bringing the knees close to the nose, keeping head and spine straight. Support yourself on the bums with the palms pressing into the ground. Pull the penis muscles as if preventing ejaculation.

अथ वज्रोलिमुद्रायाः फलकथनम् । atha vajrolimudrāyāḥ phalakathanam ।
अयं योगो योगश्रेष्ठो योगिनां मुक्तिकारणम्।अयं हितप्रदो योगो योगिनां सिद्धिदायकः॥४६
एतद्योगप्रसादेन बिन्दुसिद्धिर्भवेद्ध्रुवम् । सिद्धे बिन्दौ महायत्ने किं न सिध्यति भूतले ॥ ४७
भोगेन महता युक्तो यदि मुद्रां समाचरेत् । तथाऽपि सकला सिद्धिस्तस्य भवति निश्चितम्
॥ ४८

ayaṃ yogo yogaśreṣṭho yogināṃ muktikāraṇam । ayaṃ hitaprado

yogo yogināṃ siddhidāyakaḥ ॥ 46

etadyogaprasādena bindusiddhirbhaveddhruvam । siddhe bindau

mahāyatne kiṃ na sidhyati bhūtale ॥ 47

bhogena mahatā yukto yadi mudrāṃ samācaret । tathā'pi sakalā

siddhistasya bhavati niścitam ॥ 48

3.46-48 For men the retention of seed is an ideal mechanism to retain fitness. Man must verily strive to prevent unneeded ejaculation during copulation. The special life-giving properties of semen if it goes back inside will keep a man's body youthful and lustrous.

अथ शक्तिचालनीमुद्राकथनम् । atha śakticālanīmudrākathanam ।

मूलाधारे आत्मशक्तिः कुण्डली परदेवता । शयिता भुजगाऽऽकारा सार्धत्रिवलयाऽन्विता ॥ ४९

mūlādhāre ātmaśaktiḥ kuṇḍalī paradevatā ।

śayitā bhujagā''kārā sārdhatrivalayā'nvitā ॥ 49

3.49 The primordial energy having infinite power that we are all blessed with is normally dormant at the base of the spine. Hence it is called Kundalini, the static force in the pot shaped pelvis. Also known as the energy of the 3-1/2 syllabled sacred sound ॐ Om.

यावत्सा निद्रिता देहे तावज्जीवः पशुर्यथा । ज्ञानं न जायते तावत्कोटियोगं समभ्यसेत्॥५०

yāvatsā nidritā dehe tāvajjīvaḥ paśuryathā । jñānaṃ na jāyate tāvatkoṭiyogaṃ samabhyaset ॥ 50

3.50 This primordial energy is rarely awakened, and only partially used by the majority of human beings.

उद्घाटयेत्कवाटं च यथा कुञ्चिकया हठात् । कुण्डलिन्याः प्रबोधेन ब्रह्मद्वारं प्रभेदयेत् ॥ ५१

udghāṭayetkavāṭam ca yathā kuñcikayā haṭhāt । kuṇḍalinyāḥ

prabodhena brahmadvāraṃ prabhedayet ॥ 51

3.51 Just as light enters a door only after the key is turned in the lock and the door is thrown ajar, the practice of Hatha Yoga helps to unravel the first knot located in the pelvis, thereby stirring up the Kundalini. Only when the lid of inertia breaks does the energy begin to travel upwards at the Mooladhara Chakra.

नाभिं संवेष्ट्य वस्त्रेण न च नग्नो बहिः स्थितः । गोपनीयगृहे स्थित्वा शक्तिचालनमभ्यसेत् ॥ ५२

nābhiṃ saṃveṣṭya vastreṇa na ca nagno bahiḥ sthitaḥ |

gopanīyagṛhe sthitvā śakticālanamabhyaset || 52

3.52 Keeping one's lower private parts fully covered, and also our chest and nipples unbared, one should find a secluded spot.

Only then must the Pranayama be practiced.

वितस्तिप्रमितं दीर्घं विस्तारे चतुरङ्गुलम् । मृदुलं धवलं सूक्ष्मं वेष्टनाम्बरलक्षणम् ।
एवमम्बरयुक्तं च कटिसूत्रेण योजयेत् ॥ ५३

vitastipramitaṃ dīrghaṃ vistāre caturaṅgulam | mṛdulaṃ dhavalaṃ

sūkṣmaṃ veṣṭanāmbaralakṣaṇam | evamambarayuktaṃ ca

kaṭisūtreṇa yojayet || 53

3.53 A point to note is that the covering cloth must be soft, thin, and just enough, so as not to hamper the flow of energy.

भस्मना गात्रं संलिप्य सिद्धासनं समाचरेत् । नासाभ्यां प्राणमाकृष्य अपाने योजयेद्बलात् ॥
५४ ॥ तावदाकुञ्चयेद्गुह्यं शनैरश्विनिमुद्रया । यावद्गच्छेत्सुषुम्णायां वायुः प्रकाशयेद्धठात् ॥
५५ ॥ bhasmanā gātraṃ saṃlipya siddhāsanaṃ samācaret |

nāsābhyāṃ prāṇamākṛṣya apāne yojayedbalāt || 54

tāvadākuñcayedguhyaṃ śanairaśvinimudrayā |

yāvadgacchetsuṣumṇāyāṃ vāyuḥ prakāśayeddhaṭhāt || 55

3.54 -55 When the smell of earth can be faintly felt and the surrounding ambience has been acknowledged and is no longer of active concern.

Then the polishing of the respiratory and excretory organs by the aware breath can be begun.

Apply ashwini mudra by contracting the anal muscles and holding the breath as long as comfortable.

After a few rounds one can notice the breath becoming soft and subtle, which indicates that the Sushumna is activated.

तदा वायुप्रबन्धेन कुम्भिका च भुजङ्गिनी । बद्धश्वासस्ततो भूत्वा ऊर्ध्वमार्गं प्रपद्यते ।
शब्दद्वयं फलैकं तु योनिमुद्रां च चालयेत् ॥ ५६

tadā vāyuprabandhena kumbhikā ca bhujaṅginī | baddhaśvāsastato

bhūtvā ūrdhvamārgaṃ prapadyate | śabdadvayaṃ phalaikaṃ tu

yonimudrāṃ ca cālayet || 56

3.56 Proper practice of kumbhak i.e. strain free breath retention, when so seated in calm isolation is the key to trigger and modulate the kundalini.

विना शक्तिचालनेन योनिमुद्रा न सिध्यति । आदौ चालनमभ्यस्य योनिमुद्रां समभ्यसेत् ॥

५७ ॥ vinā śakticālanena yonimudrā na sidhyati | ādau

cālanamabhyasya yonimudrāṃ samabhyaset || 57

3.57 Having this precise breath control, in conjunction with laser like awareness of the pelvic region, is an integral component of the Yoni Mudra.

One cannot hope to achieve success in materialistic life, nor touch spiritual heights without a sound commitment to attending to all aspects of a Yogic practice.

इति ते कथितं चण्डकपाले शक्तिचालनम् । गोपनीयं प्रयत्नेन दिने दिने समभ्यसेत् ॥ ५८

iti te kathitaṃ caṇḍakapāle śakticālanam | gopanīyaṃ prayatnena

dine dine samabhyaset || 58

3.58 O lustrous and calm seeker, thus have we studied thoroughly a Yogic set that consists of awareness, breath regulation, precise muscle movement, hands positioning and body posture.

Know that real benefit accrues when it is practiced daily over several years.

अथ शक्तिचालनीमुद्रायाः फलकथनम् । atha śakticālanīmudrāyāḥ phalakathanam ।

मुद्रेयं परमा गोप्या जरामरणनाशिनी । तस्मादभ्यसनं कार्यं योगिभिः सिद्धिकाङ्क्षिभिः ॥५९

mudreyaṃ paramā gopyā jarāmaraṇanāśinī । tasmādabhyasanaṃ kāryaṃ yogibhiḥ siddhikāṅkṣibhiḥ ॥ 59

3.59 The Yogic set must be taught only to sincere seekers who qualify for the same.

नित्यं योऽभ्यसते योगी सिद्धिस्तस्य करे स्थिता ।

तस्य विग्रहसिद्धिः स्याद्रोगाणां सङ्क्षयो भवेत् ॥ ६०

nityaṃ yo'bhyasate yogī siddhistasya kare sthitā । tasya vigrahasiddhiḥ syādrogāṇāṃ saṅkṣayo bhavet ॥ 60

3.60 Man attains to a very high level of worldly understanding. He is able to keep illness and disgrace at bay, and attain to a noble standing among the successful.

अथ तडागीमुद्राकथनम् । atha taḍāgīmudrākathanam ।

उदरं पश्चिमोत्तानं कृत्वा च तडागाकृति । तडागी सा परामुद्रा जरामृत्युविनाशिनी ॥ ६१

udaraṃ paścimottānaṃ kṛtvā ca taḍāgākṛti । taḍāgī sā parāmudrā jarāmṛtyuvināśinī ॥ 61

3.61 Sitting in paschimottan asana, bring your focus to the belly, as you breathe out pull the belly in so that the curved hollow shape of an empty pond is seen.

It fires up the digestion and hence restores good health.

अथ माण्डुकीमुद्राकथनम् । atha māṇḍukīmudrākathanam ।

मुखं समुद्रितं कृत्वा जिह्वामूलं प्रचालयेत् । शनैर्ग्रसेदमृतं तन्माण्डुकीं मुद्रिकां विदुः ॥ ६२

mukhaṃ samudritaṃ kṛtvā jihvāmūlaṃ pracālayet ।

śanairgrasedamṛtaṃ tanmāṇḍukīṃ mudrikāṃ viduḥ ॥ 62

3.62 Manduki Mudra is pushing your cheeks and all areas of mouth with your tongue tip. As you make various faces, the tongue releases pent up fury from different muscles.

In this process one might get the taste of stuff stuck here and there in the teeth and gums, and when that is released, and as the muscles of the jaw release their toxins, a nectarine sensation is felt.

अथ माण्डुकीमुद्रायाः कथनम् । atha māṇḍukīmudrāyāḥ kathanam ।

वलितं पलितं नैव जायते नित्ययौवनम् । न केशे जायते पाको यः कुर्यान्नित्यमाण्डुकीम् ॥ ६३

valitaṃ palitaṃ naiva jāyate nityayauvanam । na keśe jāyate pāko

yaḥ kuryānnityamāṇḍukīm ॥ 63

3.63 Manduki helps soften us up, and as the guilt and fear slowly melt away, forgiveness dawns thereby flexibility and suppleness of the mind is retained even in old age.

Since our wits remain alert right through old age, we can apply the pun our hair haven't greyed.

अथ शाम्भवीमुद्राकथनम् । atha śāmbhavīmudrākathanam ।

नेत्राञ्जनं समालोक्य आत्मारामं निरीक्षयेत् । सा भवेच्छाम्भवी मुद्रा सर्वतन्त्रेषु गोपिता ॥ ६४

netrāñjanaṃ samālokya ātmārāmaṃ nirīkṣayet । sā

bhavecchāmbhavī mudrā sarvatantreṣu gopitā ॥ 64

3.64 Shambhavi Mudra is done by bringing the attention to the eyes, then moving the eyeballs for a moment to gaze at the junction of the eyebrows, and then closing the eyes and enjoying the sensation at the third eye.

Sometimes there isn't any feeling, at other times a strong stirring is noticed.

It gives more effect if we only observe like a witness, without analyzing, concentrating, or desiring a sensation.

As the consciousness moves over and touches the pituitary and pineal glands, their functioning improves tremendously. Only a light touch like a faint remembrance, without any tug or pull, is the correct way.

It is always more difficult to observe without judging, a fair amount of practice and discipline is required to achieve this balance.

अथ शाम्भवीमुद्रायाः फलकथनम् । atha śāmbhavīmudrāyāḥ phalakathanam
।
वेदशास्त्रपुराणानि सामान्यगणिका इव । इयं तु शाम्भवी मुद्रा गुप्ता कुलवधूरिव ॥ ६५
vedaśāstrapurāṇāni sāmānyagaṇikā iva । iyaṃ tu śāmbhavī mudrā
guptā kulavadhūriva ॥ 65
3.65 Since this is an advanced practice, be selective and careful before doing it.

Ensure you are well showered and cleanly dressed, and you have the space and time for solitude.

Remember it is not as simple as just going to school and learning some subjects and solving some equations.

It needs much more effort and preparation to welcome home a new bride and a long time, real hard work and varied experiences before she feels fully acclimatized and an honored member of the family.

स एव आदिनाथश्च स च नारायणः स्वयम् ।

स च ब्रह्मा सृष्टिकारी यो मुद्रां वेत्ति शाम्भवीम् ॥ ६६

sa eva ādināthaśca sa ca nārāyaṇaḥ svayam ।

sa ca brahmā sṛṣṭikārī yo mudrāṃ vetti śāmbhavīm ॥ 66

3.66 Shambhavi Mudra can only be learnt at the feet of a Master.
It can only be learnt when one is willing to devote effort towards
the ultimate.

सत्यं सत्यं पुनः सत्यं सत्यमुक्तं महेश्वरः ।

शाम्भवीं यो विजानीयात्स च ब्रह्म न चाऽन्यथा ॥ ६७

satyaṃ satyaṃ punaḥ satyaṃ satyamuktaṃ maheśvaraḥ ।

śāmbhavīṃ yo vijānīyātsa ca brahma na cā'nyathā ॥ 67

3.67 So has the great one said, energize and activate the third eye,
pay attention to polishing the intellect, become aware and mindful.

Only then have you lived the Truth, only then have you justified this
human birth.

अथ पञ्चधारणामुद्राकथनम् । atha pañcadhāraṇāmudrākathanam ।

कथिता शाम्भवी मुद्रा शृणुष्व पञ्चधारणाम् । धारणानि समासाद्य किं न सिध्यति भूतले ॥
६८

kathitā śāmbhavī mudrā śarṇuṣva pañcadhāraṇām । dhāraṇāni
samāsādya kiṃ na sidhyati bhūtale ॥ 68

3.68 Having heard, understood and practiced the Shambhavi, and
the asanas, mudras and bandhas, we now step into the realm of
Dharana.

अनेन नरदेहेन स्वर्गेषु गमनाऽऽगमम् । मनोगतिर्भवेत्तस्य खेचरत्वं न चाऽन्यथा ॥ ६९

anena naradehena svargeṣu gamanā''gamam ।

manogatirbhavettasya khecaratvaṃ na cā'nyathā ॥ 69

3.69 Dharana is a process to release the body's hold over the mind.

It is almost like imagination, but very potent, as the mind is brought to a focus that helps it step out of its rigid shell.

अथ पार्थिवीधारणामुद्राकथनम् । atha pārthivīdhāraṇāmudrākathanam ।
यत्तत्त्वं हरितालदेशरचितं भौमं लकाराऽन्वितं वेदास्रं कमलासनेन सहितं कृत्वा हृदि
स्थायिनम् । प्राणं तत्र विलीय पञ्चघटिकाश्चित्ताऽन्वितं धारयेद् एषा स्तम्भकरी सदा
क्षितिजयं कुर्यादधोधारणा ॥ ७०
yattattvaṃ haritāladeśaracitaṃ bhaumaṃ lakārā'nvitaṃ vedāsraṃ
kamalāsanena sahitaṃ kṛtvā hṛdi sthāyinam । prāṇaṃ tatra vilīya
pañcaghaṭikāścittā'nvitaṃ dhārayed eṣā stambhakarī sadā kṣitijayaṃ
kuryādadhodhāraṇā ॥ 70

3.70 Visualize the yellowish FORM of the solid earth. Utter its NAME "लं laṃ" to conjure the lands spreading in all the four directions.

This tangible physical element has been given the technical term Brahma in the scriptures, as it aids name and form.

Sit for a period of 24 minutes (ghati) in such contemplation for five times, this is called Adho-dharana, the lesser or simpler focus.

Then the hold of the earthly body on the mind is loosened, and one can verily plan and do tasks far greater than this frail frame would normally allow.

अथ पार्थिवीधारणामुद्रायाः फलकथनम् । atha pārthivīdhāraṇāmudrāyāḥ

phalakathanam ।
पार्थिवीधारणामुद्रां यः करोति च नित्यशः । मृत्युञ्जयः स्वयं सोऽपि स सिद्धो विचरेद्भुवि
॥ ७१

pārthivīdhāraṇāmudrāṃ yaḥ karoti ca nityaśaḥ । mṛtyuñjayaḥ

svayaṃ so'pi sa siddho vicaredbhuvi ॥ 71
3.71 The adho-dharana or simple-focus relates to earth, so is called Parthivi Dharana or Earthy Focus.

It overcomes reluctance of traveling to foreign lands, and makes one adapt to all cultures and climates.

अथाऽम्भसीधारणामुद्राकथनम् ।
शङ्खेन्दुप्रतिमं च कुन्दधवलं तत्त्वं किलालं शुभं तत्पीयूषवकारबीजसहितं युक्तं सदा
विष्णुना । प्राणं तत्र विलीय पञ्चघटिकाश्चित्ताऽन्वितं धारयेद् एषा दुःसहतापपापहरिणी
स्यादाम्भसी धारणा ॥ ७२

śaṅkhendupratimaṃ ca kundadhavalaṃ tattvaṃ kilālaṃ śubhaṃ

tatpīyūṣavakārabījasahitaṃ yuktaṃ sadā viṣṇunā ǀ prāṇaṃ tatra

vilīya pañcaghaṭikāścittā'nvitaṃ dhārayed eṣā

duḥsahatāpapāpahariṇī syādāmbhasī dhāraṇā ǁ 72

3.72 Transparent is the Water element, and it reflects light like the moon, gurgles and sounds like the conch, and is soft to touch like the jasmine flower.

The letter " वं vaṃ" is the connotation being its seed sounding syllable.

This tangible physical element has been given the technical term Vishnu in the scriptures, as it represents flow and functioning of all things and beings.

Sit for a period of 24 minutes (ghati) in such contemplation for five times over five successive days, this is called Ambhasi-dharana, the reflective or compassionate focus.

Compassion easily nullifies one's emotional distancing and thus makes one adjust and keep afloat in harsh social situations as well.

अथाऽम्भसीधारणामुद्रायाः फलकथनम् । athā'mbhasīdhāraṇāmudrāyāḥ

phalakathanam ǀ

आम्भसीं परमां मुद्रां यो जानाति स योगवित् । जले च गभीरे घोरे मरणं तस्य नो भवेत्

॥ ७३

इयं तु परमा मुद्रा गोपनीया प्रयत्नतः । प्रकाशात्सिद्धिहानिः स्यात्सत्यं वच्मि च तत्त्वतः ॥ ७४

āmbhasīṃ paramāṃ mudrāṃ yo jānāti sa yogavit | jale ca gabhīre ghore maraṇaṃ tasya no bhavet || 73

iyaṃ tu paramā mudrā gopanīyā prayatnataḥ | prakāśātsiddhihāniḥ syātsatyaṃ vacmi ca tattvataḥ || 74

3.73-74 Ambhasi-dharana or watery-dharana I.e. igniting compassion is an advanced technique.
It will prevent drowning in the turbulent societal relationships.
Compassion is not something to be explicitly expressed, it is an inner understanding alone.

अथाऽऽग्नेयीधारणामुद्राकथनम् । athā"gneyīdhāraṇāmudrākathanam |
यन्नाभिस्थितमिन्द्रगोपसदृशं बीजं त्रिकोणाऽन्वितं तत्त्वं तेजमयं प्रदीप्तमरुणं रुद्रेण यत्सिद्धिदम् । प्राणं तत्र विलीय पञ्चघटिकाश्चित्ताऽन्वितं धारयेद् एषा कालगभीरभीतिहरणी वैश्वानरी धारणा ॥ ७५

yannābhisthitamindragopasadṛśam bījaṃ trikoṇā'nvitaṃ tattvaṃ tejamayaṃ pradīptamaruṇam rudreṇa yatsiddhidam | prāṇaṃ tatra vilīya pañcaghaṭikāścittā'nvitaṃ dhārayed eṣā kālagabhīrabhītiharaṇī vaiśvānarī dhāraṇā || 75

3.75 Now we learn the Vaishvanari Dharana. That which is located at the Navel, and of the color of the indragopa flower i.e. orange, and of the shape of a triangle.

It is the lustrous fire element, of the glowing nature of the early morning sun. The semivowel रं "raṃ" is its seed representation, symbolizing the happy dancing flames.

This tangible physical element has been given the technical term Rudra in the scriptures, as it represents a total transformation of dullness, weakness, misery, and desperation. Such qualities are completely nullified and eradicated by igniting the Rudra tattva.

Sit for a period of 24 minutes (ghati) in such contemplation for at least five times (within a week).

That shall activate all the juices within, banish fears, consume constipation, and make success surface.

अथाऽऽग्नेयीधारणामुद्रायाः फलकथनम् । प्रदीप्ते ज्वलिते वह्नौ यदि पतति साधकः ।
एतन्मुद्राप्रसादेन स जीवति न मृत्युभाक् ॥ ७६

athā"gneyīdhāraṇāmudrāyāḥ phalakathanam | pradīpte jvalite

vahnau yadi patati sādhakaḥ | etanmudrāprasādena sa jīvati na

mṛtyubhāk || 76

3.76 A steady practice of this shall make the sadhak handle the fieriest situations with elan, and pressing dangers shall melt away quickly in his presence.

अथ वायवीधारणामुद्राकथनम् ।
यद्भिन्नाऽञ्जनपुञ्जसंनिभमिदं धूम्राऽवभासं परं तत्त्वं सत्त्वमयं यकारसहितं यत्रेश्वरो देवता ।
प्राणं तत्र विलीय पञ्चघटिकाश्चित्ताऽन्वितं धारयेद् एषा खे गमनं करोति यमिनां स्याद्वायवी
धारणा ॥ ७७

yadbhinnā'ñjanapuñjasaṃnibhamidam dhūmrā'vabhāsam param

tattvam sattvamayam yakārasahitam yatreśvaro devatā | prāṇam

tatra vilīya pañcaghaṭikāścittā'nvitam dhārayed eṣā khe gamanam

karoti yamināṃ syādvāyavī dhāraṇā || 77

3.77 Misty is the Air element, since it is invisible and only during fog or smoke do we physically see it and become more closely aware of air, its all-pervasiveness and begin to ponder that one can actually be free.

The semivowel यं "yaṃ" is its seed representation, symbolizing the tuning fork Y that is commonly used to move an air column.

This tangible physical element has been given the technical term Ishvar in the scriptures, as it represents lightness and flexibility a potent quality of the divine.

Sit for a period of 24 minutes (ghati) in such contemplation for minimum five times, this is called Vayavi-dharana, the moving or evolving focus.

This contemplation is most enlightening as it allows man to shed his restrictive roots and move freely like air.

अथ वायवीधारणामुद्रायाः फलकथनम् । atha vāyavīdhāraṇāmudrāyāḥ phalakathanam ।

इयं तु परमा मुद्रा जरामृत्युविनाशिनी । वायुना म्रियते नाऽपि खें गतेश्च प्रदायिनी ॥ ७८
iyaṃ tu paramā mudrā jarāmṛtyuvināśinī । vāyunā mriyate nā'pi khe gateśca pradāyinī ॥ 78

3.78 This contemplation removes the fear of closed confinement, of not being able to travel abroad, or of not being able to travel by plane or not being able to climb tall mountains where the air is thin.

शठाय भक्तिहीनाय न देया यस्य कस्यचित् ।
दत्ते च सिद्धिहानिः स्यात्सत्यं वच्मि च चण्ड ते ॥ ७९
śaṭhāya bhaktihīnāya na deyā yasya kasyacit । datte ca siddhihāniḥ syātsatyaṃ vacmi ca caṇḍa te ॥ 79

3.79 Such techniques must not be revealed to unqualified people. Unserious and callous behavior is an impediment in its learning and practice.

अथाऽऽकाशीधारणामुद्राकथनम् । athā"kāśīdhāraṇāmudrākathanam ।
यत्सिन्धौ वरशुद्धवारिसदृशं व्योमं परं भासितं तत्त्वं देवसदाशिवेन सहितं बीजं हकाराऽन्वितम् । प्राणं तत्र विलीय पञ्चघटिकाश्चित्ताऽन्वितं धारयेद् एषा मोक्षकवाटभेदनकरी कुर्यान्नभोधारणाम् ॥ ८०
yatsindhau varaśuddhavārisadṛśaṃ vyomaṃ paraṃ bhāsitam tattvaṃ devasadāśivena sahitaṃ bījaṃ hakārā'nvitam ।

prāṇaṃ tatra vilīya pañcaghaṭikāścittā'nvitaṃ dhārayed
eṣā mokṣakavāṭabhedanakarī kuryānnabhodhāraṇām ‖ 80
3.80 Deep Blue, the sight of a calm sea is the color of the ether
element.

The aspirate हं "haṃ" is how it's commonly represented,
symbolizing the feeling and exclamation of freedom.

This transcendental physical element has been given the technical
term Sadashiva in the scriptures, as it represents eternal and
continuous auspiciousness.

Sit for a period of 24 minutes (ghati) in such contemplation for five
successive times, this is called Vyoma-dharana, the expansive or
infinite focus.

Easily it leads one to deeper states of Meditation.

अथाऽऽकाशीधारणामुद्रायाः फलकथनम् । athā''kāśīdhāraṇāmudrāyāḥ
phalakathanam ।
आकाशीधारणां मुद्रां यो वेत्ति स च योगवित् ।न मृत्युर्जायते तस्य प्रलये नावसीदति ॥८१
ākāśīdhāraṇāṃ mudrāṃ yo vetti sa ca yogavit ।na mṛtyurjāyate tasya
pralaye nāvasīdati ‖ 81
3.81 One who practices the space contemplation is a true Yogi. Fear
never troubles him, nor does guilt trap him.

अथाऽश्विनीमुद्राकथनम् । athā'śvinīmudrākathanam ।
आकुञ्च्ययेद्गुदद्वारं प्रकाशयेत्पुनः पुनः । सा भवेदश्विनी मुद्रा शक्तिप्रबोधकारिणी ॥ ८२
ākuñcayedgudadvāraṃ prakāśayetpunaḥ punaḥ । sā bhavedaśvinī
mudrā śaktiprabodhakāriṇī ‖ 82
3.82 Bringing the focus at your bums, contract and dilate the anal
opening a few successive times.

This will help in proper functioning of the mooladhar chakra and infuse enthusiasm by upward flow of prana.

This technique is called Ashwini Mudra.

अथाऽश्विनीमुद्रायाः फलकथनम् । athā'śvinīmudrāyāḥ phalakathanam |
अश्विनी परमा मुद्रा गुह्यरोगविनाशिनी । बलपुष्टिकरी चैव अकालमरणं हरेत् ॥ ८३
aśvinī paramā mudrā guhyarogavināśinī | balapuṣṭikarī caiva

akālamaraṇaṃ haret ॥ 83

3.83 This Ashwini mudra is a recommended practice for quick recuperation to restore good health.
Enthusiasm is the very first step in making life enjoyable and it begins at the Root chakra.
Without any interest in life, man is almost half-dead, a vegetable existence.

अथ पशिनीमुद्राकथनम् । atha paśinīmudrākathanam |
कण्ठपृष्ठे क्षिपेत्पादौ पाशवद्दृढबन्धनम् । सैव स्यात्पाशिनी मुद्रा शक्तिप्रबोधकारिणी ॥ ८४
kaṇṭhapṛṣṭe kṣipetpādau pāśavaddṛḍhabandhanam | saiva

syātpāśinī mudrā śaktiprabodhakāriṇī ॥ 84

3.84 Pashinee Mudra or Noose Seal is an advanced yogic technique.
It involves bringing the neck between the two legs after halasan.
This mudra causes an upward flow of prana by energizing the lower chakras.

https://soulprajna.com/pashinee-mudra/

अथ पशिनीमुद्रायाः फलकथनम् । atha paśinīmudrāyāḥ phalakathanam |
पाशिनी महती मुद्रा बलपुष्टिविधायिनी । साधनीया प्रयत्नेन साधकैः सिद्धिकाङ्क्षिभिः ॥ ८५
pāśinī mahatī mudrā balapuṣṭividhāyinī | sādhanīyā prayatnena

sādhakaiḥ siddhikāṅkṣibhiḥ ॥ 85

3.85 this mudra massages the spine and strengthens the internal organs.
It is to be performed carefully under supervision by advanced practitioners only.

अथ काकीमुद्राकथनम् । atha kākīmudrākathanam ।

काकचञ्चुवदास्येन पिबेद्वायुं शनैः शनैः । काकी मुद्रा भवेदेषा सर्वरोगविनाशिनी ॥ ८६

kākacañcuvadāsyena pibedvāyuṃ śanaiḥ śanaiḥ । kākī mudrā

bhavedeṣā sarvarogavināśinī ॥ 86

3.86 The crow seal is another advanced technique. It involves sucking the air slowly through the lips pulled forward in the shape of a beak.
As the saliva mixed air goes within the body, many illnesses are prevented or get cured.

अथ काकीमुद्रायाः फलकथनम् । atha kākīmudrāyāḥ phalakathanam ।

काकीमुद्रा परा मुद्रा सर्वतन्त्रेषु गोपिता । अस्याः प्रसादमात्रेण न रोगी काकवद्भवेत् ॥ ८७

kākīmudrā parā mudrā sarvatantreṣu gopitā । asyāḥ

prasādamātreṇa na rogī kākavadbhavet ॥ 87

3.87 this kaki mudra is rarely taught as it requires enhanced lung capacity and endurance of the practitioner.

One develops a strong throat like a crow's and in turn the thyroid gland becomes more efficient, leading to prevention of many diseases.

अथ मातङ्गिनीमुद्राकथनम् । atha mātaṅginīmudrākathanam ।

कण्ठमग्ने जले स्थित्वा नासाभ्यां जलमाहरेत् ।

मुखान्निर्गमयेत्पश्चात्पुनर्वक्त्रेण चास्सहरेत् ॥ ८८

नासाभ्यां रेचयेत्पश्चात्कुर्यादेवं पुनः पुनः । मातङ्गिनी परा मुद्रा जरामृत्युविनाशिनी ॥ ८९

kaṇṭhamagne jale sthitvā nāsābhyāṃ jalamāharet |

mukhānnirgamayetpaścātpunarvaktreṇa cā"haret || 88

nāsābhyāṃ recayetpaścātkuryādevaṃ punaḥ punaḥ | mātaṅginī

parā mudrā jarāmṛtyuvināśinī || 89

3.88-89 3rd chakra.

Hear about the matangi or elephant trunk action.

Just as an elephant standing in a pool draws water in its trunk and splashes it all over its body, and does it successively a few times, to clean itself thoroughly.

So can one clasp the palms keeping middle fingers straight and joined together. Rest with the hands kept at Manipura Chakra for a few minutes. This represents the Matangini Mudra.
https://www.fitsri.com/yoga/matangi-mudra

अथ मातङ्गिनीमुद्रायाः फलकथनम् | atha mātaṅginīmudrāyāḥ

phalakathanam | विरले निर्जने देशे स्थित्वा चैकाग्रमानसः । कुर्यान्मातङ्गिनीं मुद्रां

मातङ्ग इव जायते || ९० || virale nirjane deśe sthitvā caikāgramānasaḥ |

kuryānmātaṅginīṃ mudrāṃ mātaṅga iva jāyate || 90

3.90 Matangi represents a female elephant that is known to give great pleasure to the male elephant.

यत्र यत्र स्थितो योगी सुखमत्यन्तमश्नुते । तस्मात्सर्वप्रयत्नेन साधयेन्मुद्रिकां पराम् || ९१

yatra yatra sthito yogī sukhamatyantamaśnute |

tasmātsarvaprayatnena sādhayenmudrikāṃ parām || 91

3.91 So practice this mudra in a solitary place, so that you can derive its benefits and pleasure without distraction.

अथ भुजङ्गिनीमुद्राकथनम् | atha bhujaṅginīmudrākathanam |

वक्रं किञ्चित्सुप्रसार्य चाऽनिलं गलया पिबेत् । सा भवेद्भुजङ्गी मुद्रा जरामृत्युविनाशिनी ||९२

vaktraṃ kiñcitsuprasārya cā'nilaṃ galayā pibet| sā bhavedbhujaṅgī mudrā jarāmṛtyuvināśinī ‖ 92
3.92 Bhujangini Mudra

Sitting comfortably, lean forward and stretch the neck out as you inhale through the mouth, and come back to normal posture as you exhale.

This is a snake like inhalation, and a soft hiss can be heard. It makes the spine supple and thus enhances one's fitness.
http://thelonerider.com/2019/nov/bhujangini_mudra/bhujangini_mudra.shtml

अथ भुजङ्गिनीमुद्रायाः फलकथनम् । atha bhujaṅginīmudrāyāḥ phalakathanam । यावच्च उदरे रोगा अजीर्णादि विशेषतः । तत्सर्वं नाशयेदाशु यत्र मुद्रा भुजङ्गिनी ‖ ९३ ‖ yāvacca udare rogā ajīrṇādi viśeṣataḥ | tatsarvaṃ nāśayedāśu yatra mudrā bhujaṅginī ‖ 93
3.93 the bhujangini mudra also tightens the stomach muscles, and results in a leaner frame.

अथ मुद्राणां फलकथनम् । atha mudrāṇāṃ phalakathanam |
इदं तु मुद्रापटलं कथितं चण्ड ते शुभम् । वल्लभं सर्वसिद्धानां जरामरणनाशनम् ‖ ९४
idaṃ tu mudrāpaṭalaṃ kathitaṃ caṇḍa te śubham | vallabhaṃ sarvasiddhānāṃ jarāmaraṇanāśanam ‖ 94
3.94 O calm king! Thus, have I taught in-depth the various Mudras, including Bandhaa and Dharanas.

These have an intense action on all the body parts and internal organs. Hence, they are favored by the Yoga practitioners.

शठाय भक्तिहीनाय न देयं यस्य कस्यचित् । गोपनीयं प्रयत्नेन दुर्लभं मरुतामपि ‖ ९५

śaṭhāya bhaktihīnāya na deyaṃ yasya kasyacit | gopanīyaṃ
prayatnena durlabhaṃ marutāmapi || 95
3.95 these practices must not be revealed to the cruel people, nor
to those who have no respect for the scriptures or the Lord's
glories.

The teaching must be slow and methodical over several days. The
progress of the participants and their understanding must be
carefully noted before beginning a new technique.

It takes a serious learner much effort to actually ingrain this
knowledge and activate his chakras properly.

ऋजवे शान्तचित्ताय गुरुभक्तिपराय च । कुलीनाय प्रदातव्यं भोगमुक्तिप्रदायकम् ॥ ९६
rjave śāntacittāya gurubhaktiparāya ca | kulīnāya pradātavyaṃ
bhogamuktipradāyakam || 96
3.96 the devotion and faith of the seeker must also be watched and
nurtured, it makes sense only when the student grows in these
values and becomes a peace-loving and Nature respecting
individual.

मुद्राणां पटलं ह्येतत्सर्वव्याधिविनाशनम् । नित्यमभ्यासशीलस्य जठराग्निविवर्धनम् ॥ ९७
mudrāṇāṃ paṭalam hyetatsarvavyādhivināśanam |
nityamabhyāsaśīlasya jaṭharāgnivivardhanam || 97
3.97 the feverish desires of man can well be calmed and directed
towards productive efforts.

His emotions of greed and jealousy can also be tamed likewise.

न तस्य जायते मृत्युर्नास्य जरादिकं तथा । नाग्निजलभयं तस्य वायोरपि कुतो भयम् ॥ ९८
na tasya jāyate mṛtyurnāsya jarādikam tathā | nāgnijalabhayam
tasya vāyorapi kuto bhayam || 98

3.98 Man overcomes his destructive tendencies, remains self-dependent even in old age.

His usage of fire, water and air is also conservative, and his wastage of natural resources is minimal.

कासः श्वासः प्लीहा कुष्ठं श्लेष्मरोगाश्च विंशतिः । मुद्राणां साधनाच्चैव विनश्यन्ति न संशयः

॥ ९९ ॥ kāsaḥ śvāsaḥ plīhā kuṣṭham śleṣmarogāśca viṃśatiḥ ।

mudrāṇāṃ sādhanāccaiva vinaśyanti na saṃśayaḥ ॥ 99
3.99 more than 20 common and rare illnesses can be prevented and cured by a regular practice of the Mudras-Bandhas-Dharanas.

बहुना किमिहोक्तेन सारं वच्मि च चण्ड ते । नास्ति मुद्रासमं किञ्चित्सिद्धिदं क्षितिमण्डले

॥ १०० ॥ bahunā kimihoktena sāram vacmi ca caṇḍa te । nāsti

mudrāsamam kiñcitsiddhidam kṣitimaṇḍale ॥ 100
3.100 Remember o great king! These practices are relatively easy and doable for most members of society, thus they must verily be learnt and dutifully practiced.

॥ इति श्रीघेरण्डसंहितायां घेरण्डचण्डकापालिसंवादे घटस्थयोगप्रकरणे
मुद्राप्रयोगो नाम तृतीयोपदेशः ॥ iti śrīgheraṇḍasaṃhitāyāṃ
gheraṇḍacaṇḍakāpālisaṃvāde ghaṭasthayogaprakaraṇe
mudrāprayogo nāma tṛtīyopadeśaḥ ॥
Here ends the 3rd chapter.

4 Inward U turn - Pratyahara प्रत्याहारप्रयोगो नाम चतुर्थोपदेशः

घेरण्ड उवाच । gheraṇḍa uvāca । अथातः सम्प्रवक्ष्यामि प्रत्याहारमनुत्तमम् । यस्य विज्ञानमात्रेण कामादिरिपुनाशनम् ॥ १ ॥ athātaḥ sampravakṣyāmi

pratyāhāramanuttamam । yasya vijñānamātreṇa

kāmādiripunāśanam ॥ 1

4.1 We learn a very subtle and potent technique to keep lust and arrogance at bay. It is called pratyahara = prati-ahara = that which shuts off sensual traps.

यतो यतो निश्चरति मनश्चञ्चलमस्थिरम् । ततस्ततो नियम्यैतदात्मन्येव वशं नयेत् ॥ २

yato yato niścarati manaścañcalamasthiram । tatastato

niyamyaitadātmanyeva vaśaṃ nayet ॥ 2

4.2 When the thoughts fluctuate, being pulled strongly by the senses or triggered by memory, just become aware of the phenomenon. When you become aware that you are being baited, that is the first step to overcome the bait.

यत्र यत्र गता दृष्टिर्मनस्तत्र प्रगच्छति । ततः प्रत्याहरेदेतदात्मन्येव वशं नयेत् ॥ ३

yatra yatra gatā dṛṣṭirmanastatra pragacchati । tataḥ

pratyāharedetadātmanyeva vaśaṃ nayet ॥ 3

4.3 When the eyes flirt, just become aware of it.

पुरस्कारं तिरस्कारं सुश्राव्यं दुःश्रुतं तथा । मनस्तस्मान्नियम्यैतदात्मन्येव वशं नयेत् ॥ ४

puraskāraṃ tiraskāraṃ suśrāvyaṃ duḥśrutaṃ tathā ।

manastasmānniyamyaitadātmanyeva vaśaṃ nayet ॥ 4

4.4 Heaps of flattery or loads of shame, kind remarks or terrible tongues, just become aware that it is happening, and in that awareness the storm weakens. The sounds lose their crushing hold.

शीतं वापि तथा चोष्णं यन्मनःस्पर्शयोगतः । तस्मात्प्रत्याहरेदेतदात्मन्येव वशं नयेत्॥५

śītaṃ vāpi tathā coṣṇaṃ yanmanaḥsparśayogataḥ |

tasmātpratyāharedetadātmanyeva vaśaṃ nayet || 5

4.5 When the skin says it's too cold or too hot, just become aware of it, and the mind settles down without complaining for heater or ac.

सुगन्धे वाऽपि दुर्गन्धे घ्राणेषु जायते मनः । तस्मात्प्रत्याहरेदेतदात्मन्येव वशं नयेत् ॥ ६

sugandhe vā'pi durgandhe ghrāṇeṣu jāyate manaḥ |

tasmātpratyāharedetadātmanyeva vaśaṃ nayet || 6

4.6 When you are attracted by strong smells, whether pleasant or unpleasant, just become aware - O I am being hijacked by the odors, and their pull will weaken.

मधुराम्लकतिक्तादिरसं गतं यदा मनः । तस्मात्प्रत्याहरेदेतदात्मन्येव वशं नयेत् ॥ ७

madhurāmlakatiktādirasaṃ gataṃ yadā manaḥ |

tasmātpratyāharedetadātmanyeva vaśaṃ nayet || 7

4.7 Notice your tongue if it tricks you into eating more than usual, also become alert when it shuns food saying it is insipid. These are the moments when you apply Pratyahara to avoid being sunk by your senses.

॥ इति श्रीघेरण्डसंहितायां घेरण्डचण्डसंवादे घटस्थयोगे प्रत्याहारप्रयोगो नाम चतुर्थोपदेशः ॥ iti śrīgheraṇḍasaṃhitāyāṃ gheraṇḍacaṇḍasaṃvāde ghaṭasthayoge pratyāhāraprayogo nāma caturthopadeśaḥ || Here ends the 4th teaching.

5 Breath Regulation-Pranayama प्राणायामप्रयोगो नाम पञ्चमोपदेशः

घेरण्ड उवाच । gheraṇḍa uvāca ।

अथाऽतः संप्रवक्ष्यामि प्राणायामस्य यद्विधिम् । यस्य साधनमात्रेण देवतुल्यो भवेन्नरः ॥ १

athā'taḥ sampravakṣyāmi prāṇāyāmasya yadvidhim | yasya

sādhanamātreṇa devatulyo bhavennaraḥ ॥ 1

5.1 And now we shall investigate the mechanism of breath. We shall make an in-depth study of ways and means to regulate the breath, so that our lung capacity rises significantly. We shall see how proper breathing can expand our brain and help the growth of neurons, so that our intellect can reach gigantic heights.

आदौ स्थानं तथा कालं मिताऽहारं तथापरम् ।

नाडीशुद्धि ततः पश्चात्प्राणायामं च साधयेत् ॥ २

ādau sthānaṃ tathā kālaṃ mitā'hāraṃ tathāparam | nāḍīśuddhiṃ

tataḥ paścātprāṇāyāmaṃ ca sādhayet ॥ 2

5.2 four factors influencing Pranayama are place, season, food and breath

Breath practice has some essential ground rules. These are

- a **place** where one feels accepted, light and easy. That means an ambience and atmosphere where our emotions are not under strain, and we feel a sense of freedom.
- **Season** or time of day which is as per our temperament. When our senses are alert, when our body is not tired, when we do not have other targets bothering us.
- it also goes without saying that we must not be hungry nor overfed nor have just eaten **food** that is still creating sensations in our mouth and stomach.
- lastly as we go deeper into our breath practice, we shall also realise the importance of not having blocked nose, cold and cough, sinuses or headache when we sit for our Pranayama.

Regarding Place अथ स्थाननिर्णयः ।

दूरदेशे तथाऽरण्ये राजधान्यां जनान्तिके । योगारम्भं न कुर्वीत कृतश्चेत्सिद्धिहा भवेत् ॥ ३

dūradeśe tathā'raṇye rājadhānyāṃ janāntike | yogārambhaṃ na kurvīta kṛtaścetsiddhihā bhavet || 3

5.3 Place should be one that is clean, free from disturbing noises, and that is neither suffocating nor windy.

अविश्वासं दूरदेशे अरण्ये रक्षिवर्जितम् । लोकारण्ये प्रकाशश्च तस्मात्त्रीणि विवर्जयेत् ॥ ४

aviśvāsaṃ dūradeśe araṇye rakṣivarjitam | lokāraṇye prakāśaśca tasmāttrīṇi vivarjayet || 4

5.4 nor should the place be unfriendly or stressful in any way.

सुदेशे धार्मिके राज्ये सुभिक्षे निरुपद्रवे । तत्रैकं कुटिरं कृत्वा प्राचीरैः परिवेष्टितम् ॥ ५

sudeśe dhārmike rājye subhikṣe nirupadrave | tatraikaṃ kuṭiraṃ kṛtvā prācīraiḥ pariveṣṭitam || 5

5.5 in a loving environment, where meals are served on time, and people do not make fun, which is relatively free of movements, one may spread one's mat.

वापीकूपतडागं च प्राचीरमध्यवर्ति च । नात्युच्चं नातिनिम्नं च कुटिरं कीटवर्जितम् ॥ ६

vāpīkūpataḍāgaṃ ca prācīramadhyavarti ca | nātyuccaṃ nātinimnaṃ ca kuṭiraṃ kīṭavarjitam || 6

5.6 ensure that the mat is proper in thickness, does not slide easily, has joint support and of enough size to lie down comfortably.

सम्यग्गोमयलिप्तं च कुटिरं तत्र निर्मितम् । एवं स्थाने हि गुप्ते च प्राणायामं समभ्यसेत् ॥७

samyaggomayaliptaṃ ca kuṭiraṃ tatra nirmitam | evaṃ sthāne hi gupte ca prāṇāyāmaṃ samabhyaset || 7

5.7 Make adequate arrangements for mosquito and flies' control so that such botherations are kept to a minimum. However, use only natural disinfectants and avoid any harmful chemical-based formulations.

The place having been secured, let us now see regarding the suitability of time and season.

Regarding Time and Season अथ कालनिर्णयः ।

हेमन्ते शिशिरे ग्रीष्मे वर्षायां च ऋतौ तथा । योगारम्भं न कुर्वीत कृते योगो हि रोगदः ॥८

hemante śiśire grīṣme varṣāyāṃ ca ṛtau tathā | yogārambhaṃ na

kurvīta kṛte yogo hi rogadaḥ ॥ 8

5.8 Know that the temperature must be convenient for the practitioner. Some of us like it a bit cool, others prefer a warmer climate. So make the air-conditioning accordingly or begin your practice in the appropriate season of the year. Avoid seasons when there are dust storms, hot winds or chilly weather.

Secondly the time of day must also suit you the practitioner. Some of us are more alive early morning, others feel alert and fit later in the day. In any case choose a time of day when you feel really fit and ready for Yogic practice.

वसन्ते शरदि प्रोक्तं योगारम्भं समाचरेत् । तथा योगी भवेत्सिद्धो रोगान्मुक्तो भवेद्ध्रुवम् ॥९

vasante śaradi proktaṃ yogārambhaṃ samācaret | tathā yogī

bhavetsiddho rogānmukto bhaveddhruvam ॥ 9

5.9 Never start doing it just for the heck of it, nor to impress someone, and certainly not when you are bodily tired or mentally fatigued.

चैत्रादिफाल्गुनान्ते च माघादिफाल्गुनान्तिके । द्वौ द्वौ मासावृतुभागावनुभावश्चतुश्चतुः ॥१०

caitrādiphālgunānte ca māghādiphālgunāntike | dvau dvau

māsāvṛtubhāgāvanubhāvaścatuścatuḥ ॥ 10

5.10 The weather and climate play an important role. There are six seasons of two months each, beginning with chaitra in April and ending with phalguna in March, during the course of one year.

Even though there are the six seasons, we experience practically only three, namely extreme summer, extreme winter, and a moderate third.

वसन्तश्चैत्रवैशाखौ ज्येष्ठाषाढौ च ग्रीष्मकौ । वर्षा श्रावणभाद्राभ्यां शरदाश्विनकार्तिकौ ।
मार्गपौषौ च हेमन्तः शिशिरो माघफाल्गुनौ ॥ ११

vasantaścaitravaiśākhau jyeṣṭhāṣāḍhau ca grīṣmakau | varṣā

śrāvaṇabhādrābhyāṃ śaradāśvinakārtikau | mārgapauṣau ca

hemantaḥ śiśiro māghaphālgunau || 11

5.11 Names of seasons and months are listed. However the key is not to memorize the names, rather to associate and remember one's own moods and mindsets in each season from experience, and then notice if such a mood is springing up during your practice, and shrug it aside without becoming ruffled.

अनुभावं प्रवक्ष्यामि ऋतूनां च यथोदितम् । माघादिमाधवान्तेषु वसन्तानुभवं विदुः ॥ १२
चैत्रादि चाषाढान्तं च निदाघानुभवं विदुः । आषाढादि चाश्विनान्तं प्रावृषानुभवं विदुः ॥१३
भाद्रादिमार्गशीर्षान्तं शरदोऽनुभवं विदुः । कार्तिकादिमाघमासान्तं हेमन्तानुभवं विदुः ।
मार्गादिचतुरो मासाञ्छिशिरानुभवं विदुः ॥ १४ ॥ anubhāvaṃ pravakṣyāmi

ṛtūnāṃ ca yathoditam | māghādimādhavānteṣu vasantānubhavaṃ

viduḥ || 12 || caitrādi cāṣāḍhāntaṃ ca nidāghānubhavaṃ viduḥ |

āṣāḍhādi cāśvināntaṃ prāvṛṣānubhavaṃ viduḥ || 13 ||

bhādrādimārgaśīrṣāntaṃ śarado'nubhavaṃ viduḥ |

kārtikādimāghamāsāntaṃ hemantānubhavaṃ viduḥ | mārgādicaturo

māsāñśiśirānubhavaṃ viduḥ || 14

5.12 - 5.14 Each season leaves an imprint on the psyche. Where and when we were born and spent our childhood, has already shaped not just our anatomy, but has left deep impressions of likes and dislikes regarding the climate and humidity. Such preferences must not be ignored, rather for one's Yoga practice to yield fruit, one should ensure equitable and likeable environment as per one's temperament.

Remember that even today, sportsmen have always dominated on home turf, and when they go to play in a distant land they first take some time to acclimatise themselves there.

वसन्ते वापि शरदि योगारम्भं समाचरेत्।तदा योगी भवेत्सिद्धो विनाऽऽयासेन कथ्यते॥१५

vasante vāpi śaradi yogārambhaṃ samācaret|tadā yogī

bhavetsiddho vinā''yāsena kathyate ‖ 15

5.15 Also some of us prefer well lit rooms, while others like dimly lit or even darker ambience for a more fulfilling practice. Such considerations must be adhered to.

Regarding Food अथ मिताहारः ।

मिताहारं विना यस्तु योगारम्भं तु कारयेत् । नानारोगो भवेत्तस्य किञ्चिद्योगो न सिध्यति

‖ १६ ‖ mitāhāraṃ vinā yastu yogārambhaṃ tu kārayet | nānārogo

bhavettasya kiñcidyogo na sidhyati ‖ 16

5.16 one must ensure diet that is wholesome and nutritious, mentally fulfilling and tasty. And from self experience one must avoid or regulate foodstuffs that have caused one to fall ill, whether a minor stomach ache or body ache, or an aggravating indigestion. Without such precaution no Yoga practice can ever give the desired result.

Know that timely and proper diet suitable for oneself has to be ensured and adhered to as a prerequisite for Yogic practice.

शाल्यन्नं यवपिष्टं वा गोधूमपिष्टकं तथा । मुद्गं माषचणकादि शुभ्रं च तुषवर्जितम् ॥ १७

śālyannaṃ yavapiṣṭaṃ vā godhūmapiṣṭakaṃ tathā | mudgaṃ

māṣacaṇakādi śubhraṃ ca tuṣavarjitam ‖ 17

5.17 Depending on where the practitioner lives, local grains must be an important part. Foreign foods or foods from distant lands must be kept to a minimum since they do not have the biochemical composition that one can readily digest. Nature has made a system to match the chemistry locally, more or less like a life partner that most prefer to be from one's own fraternity or race and religion so that she understands the protocols and can support the emotions.

पटोलं पनसं मानं कक्कोलं च शुकाशकम् । द्राढिकां कर्कटीं रम्भां डुम्बरीं कण्टकण्टकम् ॥ १८ ॥ आमरम्भां बालरम्भां रम्भादण्डं च मूलकम्।वार्ताकीं मूलकमृद्धिं योगी भक्षणमाचरेत्॥१९ ॥ paṭolaṃ panasaṃ mānaṃ kakkolaṃ ca śukāśakam | drāḍhikāṃ karkaṭīṃ rambhāṃ ḍumbarīṃ kaṇṭakaṇṭakam ॥ 18

āmarambhāṃ bālarambhāṃ rambhādaṇḍaṃ ca mūlakam | vārtākīṃ mūlakamṛddhiṃ yogī bhakṣaṇamācaret ॥ 19

5.18 - 19 Regarding fruits and medicinal herbs also, be strict in checking if these are locally grown. Most of us are actually unable to digest foreign foods that are similar but have slightly different mix of proteins. Our gut and digestive system can notice these minor differences, while our tongue cannot. So similar fruits from distant lands will fail to get assimilated since our physiochemistry is not meant for it. The result is some of us keep falling ill regularly, or otherwise have a weak disposition.

In some cases, one needs to change our locale or city because where we stay there the water doesn't suit us.

These are common hurdles, but only a strong willed and aware practitioner can apply changes to diet.

बालशाकं कालशाकं तथा पटोलपत्रकम् पञ्चशाकं प्रशंसीयाद्वास्तूकं हिलमोचिकाम् ॥ २०
bālaśākaṃ kālaśākaṃ tathā paṭolapatrakam |

pañcaśākaṃ praśaṃsīyādvāstūkaṃ hilamocikām ॥ 20
5.20 Regarding vegetables, know that their nutrition shelf-life is rather short, while their physical shelf-life is much longer. The

vitamins in veggies diminish rapidly as the days pass, so unless one is eating vegetables that were plucked from the field not more than 2 days past, is really not getting enough nutrition. After one week of plucking, only roughage and a bit of taste remain, medically it is proven that such veggies have no prana.

शुद्धं सुमधुरं स्निग्धमुदरार्धविवर्जितम् । भुज्यते सुरसं प्रीत्या मिताहारमिमं विदुः ॥ २१

śuddhaṃ sumadhuraṃ snigdhamudarārdhavivarjitam | bhujyate

surasaṃ prītyā mitāharamimaṃ viduḥ || 21

5.21 Hear now regarding the taste buds and how much importance each has on the anatomy.

Sweet foodstuffs that have liquid content like kheer, dalia, semia, etc should be taken in sufficient quantity as it is the brain's primary requirement.

अन्नेन पूरयेदर्धं तोयेन तु तृतीयकम् । उदरस्य तुरीयांशं संरक्षेद्वायुचारणे ॥ २२

annena pūrayedardhaṃ toyena tu tṛtīyakam | udarasya turīyāṃśaṃ

saṃrakṣedvāyucāraṇe || 22

5.22 Grains, salads, vegetables and solid foods can be taken in enough measure, supported ably by soups, juices and liquids. However, a part of the stomach should be kept empty, in other words do not over eat, never stuff yourself. Understand that the digestive mechanism needs some space to mix the enzymes and turn around the food in the stomach so that each portion gets metabolised.

Just as a washing machine can clean much better if it ain't stuffed, and a steam cooker can cook thoroughly if there is space for steam movement within.

कद्वह्लं लवणं तिक्तं भृष्टं च दधि तक्रकम् । शाकोत्कटं तथा मद्यं तालं च पनसं तथा ॥ २३
कुलत्थं मसूरं पाण्डुं कूष्माण्डं शाकदण्डकम् । तुम्बीकोलकपित्थं च कण्टबिल्वं पलाशकम्
॥ २४ ॥ कदम्बं जम्बीरं बिम्बं लकुचं लशुनं विषम् ।कामरङ्गं पियालं च

हिङ्गुशाल्मलिकेमुकम्॥ २५ ॥ kaṭvamlaṃ lavaṇaṃ tiktaṃ bhṛṣṭaṃ ca dadhi takrakam | śākotkaṭaṃ tathā madyaṃ tālaṃ ca panasaṃ tathā || 23

kulatthaṃ masūraṃ pāṇḍuṃ kūṣmāṇḍaṃ śākadaṇḍakam | tumbīkolakapitthaṃ ca kaṇṭabilvaṃ palāśakam || 24

kadambaṃ jambīraṃ bimbaṃ lakucaṃ laśunaṃ viṣam | kāmaraṅgaṃ piyālaṃ ca hiṅguśālmalikemukam || 25

5.23 - 25 Some prohibited foods are listed. However the purpose is not to blindly skip all these items, rather for the practitioner to be made aware that one must be choosy and selective and have a diet plan.

Also the Rishi says that foods that cause burning in the mouth or stomach, foods that make one uneasy later, or foods that are known to be disease causing by society at large must be altogether shunned.

योगारम्भे वर्जयेच्च पथस्त्रीवह्निसेवनम् ॥ २६

yogārambhe varjayecca pathastrīvahnisevanam || 26

5.26 when a yoga plan is started, keep your out of town travel to a minimum. Neither the diet nor the ambience can be replicated during sojourn, and even if one or two days are skipped in a month, the body and mind cannot attain to higher planes.

Another thing to avoid during the yoga programme is romantic thrills and lust provoking engagements.

Also avoid engaging orhaving lengthy conversations with maidservants or teenagers.

नवनीतं घृतं क्षीरं गुडं शर्करादि चैक्षवम् । पक्वरम्भां नारिकेलं दाडिम्बमशिवासवम् । द्राक्षां तु लवनीं धात्रीं रसमम्लविवर्जितम् ॥ २७ ॥ navanītaṃ ghṛtaṃ kṣīraṃ guḍaṃ śarkarādi caikṣavam | pakvarambhāṃ nārikelaṃ

dāḍimbamaśivāsavam | drākṣāṃ tu lavanīṃ dhātrīṃ
rasamamlavivarjitam || 27
5.27
On the other hand, meaningful company or satsang or listening to spiritual discourses is highly recommended. It evokes sweetness in the soul, calms the brain, and keeps the senses clean.

एलाजातिलवङ्गं च पौरुषं जम्बुजाम्बलम् । हरीतकीं खर्जूरं च योगी भक्षणमाचरेत् ॥ २८
लघुपाकं प्रियं स्निग्धं तथा धातुप्रपोषणम् ।मनोऽभिलषितं योग्यं योगी भोजनमाचरेत्॥ २९
काठिन्यं दुरितं पूतिमुष्णं पर्युषितं तथा। अतिशीतं चाति चोष्णं भक्ष्यं योगी विवर्जयेत्॥३०

elājātilavaṅgaṃ ca pauruṣaṃ jambujāmbalam | harītakīṃ kharjūraṃ

ca yogī bhakṣaṇamācaret ||28|| laghupākaṃ priyaṃ snigdhaṃ tathā

dhātupraposaṇam | mano'bhilaṣitaṃ yogyaṃ yogī bhojanamācaret ||

29 || kāṭhinyaṃ duritaṃ pūtimuṣṇaṃ paryuṣitaṃ tathā | atiśītaṃ

cāti coṣṇaṃ bhakṣyaṃ yogī vivarjayet || 30
5.28 -30
Always ensure a personal diet plan according to one's constitution. Also make sure to include food items one had as a child, since our physiochemistry has developed accordingly.

So while curds suit one individual, they are highly toxic for another, hence shouldn't be forced on both.

In this regard an expert nadi-pariksha doctor and one's own taste buds and past experience will come in handy.

Remember to take notes whenever you fell sick, uneasy or in pain, and jot down the things you ate just before, and over the past two days. A major clue will pop up, and next time avoid or go slow on those food stuffs. Secondly, also remember where you ate and who had cooked the food, because their aura and thoughts might also have endangered the food.

These things a practitioner must learn early on and improve upon for smoothness in Yoga practice.

प्रातःस्नानोपवासादिकायक्लेशविधिं तथा । एकाहारं निराहारं यामान्ते च न कारयेत् ॥ ३१

prātaḥsnānopavāsādikāyakleśavidhiṃ tathā | ekāhāraṃ nirāhāraṃ yāmānte ca na kārayet ॥ 31

5.31 The system of bathing, washing hands and feet, change of soiled or perspiration filled clothes, should also be attended to for enhancement in results.

एवं विधिविधानेन प्राणायामं समाचरेत् । आरम्भे प्रथमे कुर्यात्क्षीराज्यं नित्यभोजनम् । मध्याह्ने चैव सायाह्ने भोजनद्वयमाचरेत् ॥ ३२ ॥ evaṃ vidhividhānena prāṇāyāmaṃ samācaret | ārambhe prathame kuryātkṣīrājyaṃ nityabhojanam | madhyāhne caiva sāyāhne bhojanadvayamācaret ॥ 32

5.32 It will help a lot if for a few days we add fresh cow's milk and ghee in our diet, and have large meals twice daily, once around noon say 11am to 1pm, and another around evening say between 530 to 730pm.

That is sufficient regarding the diet and meal times. Now we move on to prerequisites for breath practice.

अथ नाडीशुद्धिः । atha nāḍīśuddhiḥ । कुशासने मृगाजिने व्याघ्राजिने च कम्बले । स्थलासने समासीनः प्राङ्मुखो वाप्युदङ्मुखः । नाडीशुद्धिं समासाद्य प्राणायामं समभ्यसेत् ॥ ३३ ॥ kuśāsane mṛgājine vyāghrājine ca kambale | sthalāsane samāsīnaḥ prāṅmukho vāpyudaṅmukhaḥ | nāḍīśuddhiṃ samāsādya prāṇāyāmaṃ samabhyaset ॥ 33

5.33 Choose a flat ground or hard floor. Spread your mat along the East West axis.

Ensure proper size, texture and firmness of the mattress.

One must also have a clean bedsheet for lying down and a shawl for covering oneself when resting.

These things are very crucial to begin the practice.

Now we must start the Nadi Shodhana pranayama.

चण्डकापालिरुवाच । caṇḍakāpāliruvāca ।
नाडीशुद्धिं कथं कुर्यान्नाडीशुद्धिस्तु कीदृशी । तत्सर्वं श्रोतुमिच्छामि तद्वदस्व दयानिधे॥ ३४
nāḍīśuddhiṃ kathaṃ kuryānnāḍīśuddhistu kīdṛśī । tatsarvaṃ

śrotumicchāmi tadvadasva dayānidhe ॥ 34
5.34 The brilliant disciple eagerly asked.
O respected master! O fountain of compassion! What is Nadi Shodhana? How must we do it? Please guide me step by step. I am eager to learn and follow the correct method.

घेरण्ड उवाच । gheraṇḍa uvāca । मलाकुलासु नाडीषु मारुतो नैव गच्छति ।
प्राणायामः कथं सिध्येत्तत्त्वज्ञानं कथं भवेत् । तस्मादादौ नडीशुद्धिं प्राणायामं ततोऽभ्यसेत्

॥ ३५ ॥ malākulāsu nāḍīṣu māruto naiva gacchati । prāṇāyāmaḥ

kathaṃ sidhyettattvajñānaṃ kathaṃ bhavet । tasmādādau

naḍīśuddhiṃ prāṇāyāmaṃ tato'bhyaset ॥ 35
5.35 The great master replied. Our body is composed of two types of tubes for the flow of air. One is the physical wind pipe and lungs with its associated paraphernalia needed for respiration.

The other is the subtle group of channels, know as the nadis.

Earlier when we did the Shatkarma, we purified the physical tubular structure and anatomy.

But now we need to cleanse, align, and invigorate our subtle being, and that is what is Nadi Shodhana.

नाडीशुद्धिर्द्विधा प्रोक्ता समनुर्निर्मनुस्तथा । बीजेन समनुं कुर्यान्निर्मनुं धौतिकर्मणा ॥ ३६

nāḍīśuddhirdvidhā proktā samanurnirmanustathā | bījena samanuṃ kuryānnirmanuṃ dhautikarmaṇā || 36

5.36 Nadi Shodhana is done by two means. One is by the use of Bija mantra or seed sounds, known as Sam-anu. (using specific sound frequencies to work along with the atoms of the brain to energize the neural networks). Once the neural networks are strengthened and created anew, they begin to have a positive impact on the subtle nadis and the chakras.

The other is by physical processes of working on the anatomy, known as Nir-m-anu (where the neural pathways are not modified).

धौतिकर्म पुरा प्रोक्तं षड्कर्मसाधने यथा । शृणुष्व समनुं चण्ड नाडीशुद्धिर्यथा भवेत् ॥ ३७

dhautikarma purā proktaṃ ṣaṭkarmasādhane yathā | śarṇuṣva samanuṃ caṇḍa nāḍīśuddhiryathā bhavet || 37

5.37 The latter we have learnt and practiced in our Shatkarma body cleansing processes.

Now we learn the Samanu or brain energising techniques.

उपविश्यासने योगी पद्मासनं समाचरेत् । गुर्वादिन्यासनं कुर्याद्यथैव गुरुभाषितम् । नाडीशुद्धि प्रकुर्वीत प्राणायामविशुद्धये ॥ ३८ ॥ upaviśyāsane yogī

padmāsanaṃ samācaret | gurvādinyāsanaṃ kuryādyathaiva gurubhāṣitam | nāḍīśuddhiṃ prakurvīta prāṇāyāmaviśuddhaye || 38

5.38 Sit in Padmasana or a comfortable posture where your spine is erect, shoulders are relaxed and face has a gentle smile.

Now chant your Guru Mantra, using appropriate words eulogize and praise your guru, thank him and seek his grace.

This is the first step of the Nadi Shodhana.

वायुबीजं ततो ध्यात्वा धूम्रवर्णं सतेजसम् । चन्द्रेण पूरयेद्वायुं बीजषोडशकैः सुधीः ॥ ३९

चतुःषष्ट्या मात्रया च कुम्भकेनैव धारयेत् । द्वात्रिंशन्मात्रया वायुं सूर्यनाड्या च रेचयेत् ॥

४० ॥ vāyubījaṃ tato dhyātvā dhūmravarṇaṃ satejasam | candreṇa

pūrayedvāyuṃ bījaṣoḍaśakaiḥ sudhīḥ ॥ 39 ॥ catuḥṣaṣṭyā mātrayā

ca kumbhakenaiva dhārayet | dvātriṃśanmātrayā vāyuṃ sūryanāḍyā

ca recayet ॥ 40

5.39 -40 Then assume the position of alternate nostril breathing
using the right hand.

We start breathing in from the left nostril, and then breath out from
the right nostril.

Focus the mind on the air element. As an analogy to quickly bring
your focus to the wind, remember the greyish smoke swirling in a
gentle breeze.

0) keep your attention at anahata the heart center.
1) Chant the sound yam यं ,
2) Inhale from the left side for a count of 16
3) hold the breath for a count of 64, and
4) breath out from the right side for a count of 32.

You may repeat this a few times say (2 or 3 times) to get the proper
sequence, timing and rhythm.

नाभिमूलाद्वह्निमुत्थाप्य ध्यायेत्तेजोऽवनीयुतम् । वह्निबीजषोडशेन सूर्यनाड्या च पूरयेत् ॥

४१ ॥ चतुःषष्ट्या मात्रया च कुम्भकेनैव धारयेत् । द्वात्रिंशन्मात्रया वायुं शशिनाड्या च

रेचयेत् ॥ ४२ ॥ nābhimūlādvahnimutthāpya dhyāyettejo'vanīyutam |

vahnibījaṣoḍaśena sūryanāḍyā ca pūrayet ॥ 41 ॥ catuḥṣaṣṭyā

mātrayā ca kumbhakenaiva dhārayet | dvātriṃśanmātrayā vāyuṃ śaśināḍyā ca recayet || 42

5.41 -42 Then assume the position of alternate nostril breathing using the right hand.

We start breathing in from the left nostril, and then breath out from the right nostril.

Focus the mind on the fire element. As an analogy to quickly bring your focus to the fiery glow, remember the morning sun rising through a cloudy sky.

0) keep your attention at manipura the navel center.
1) Chant the sound yam रं ,
2) Inhale from the left side for a count of 16
3) hold the breath for a count of 64, and
4) breath out from the right side for a count of 32.
You may repeat this a few times say (2 or 3 times) to get the proper sequence, timing and rhythm.

नासाग्रे शशधृग्बिम्बं ध्यात्वा ज्योत्स्नासमन्वितम् । ठं बीजं षोडशेनैव इडया पूरयेन्मरुत् ॥ ४३ ॥ चतुःषष्ठ्या मात्रया च वं बीजेनैव धारयेत् । अमृतं प्लावितं ध्यात्वा नाडीधौतं विभावयेत् । लकारेण द्वात्रिंशेन दृढं भाव्यं विरेचयेत् ॥ ४४ ॥ nāsāgre śaśadhṛgbimbaṃ dhyātvā jyotsnāsamanvitam | ṭhaṃ bījaṃ ṣoḍaśenaiva iḍayā pūrayenmarut || 43 || catuḥṣaṣṭyā mātrayā ca vaṃ bījenaiva dhārayet | amṛtaṃ plāvitaṃ dhyātvā nāḍīdhautaṃ vibhāvayet | lakāreṇa dvātriṃśena dṛḍhaṃ bhāvyaṃ virecayet || 44

5.43 -44 Assume the position of alternate nostril breathing using the right hand.

We start breathing in from the left nostril, and then breath out from the right nostril.

Focus the mind at the tip of the nose. As an analogy to quickly bring your focus to the nose, remember the soothing silvery moonlight reflecting in the water as you see your nose clearly.

0) keep your attention at the tip of the nose.
1) Chant the sound yam ठं ,
2) Inhale from the left side for a count of 16
3) hold the breath for a count of 64, and
4) breath out from the right side for a count of 32.

You may repeat this a few times say (2 or 3 times) to get the proper sequence, timing and rhythm.

Now Focus the mind on the water element. As an analogy to quickly bring your focus imagine the silvery moonlight shimmering in the water running through your entire body.

0) keep your attention at swadhisthana the genital center.
1) Chant the sound yam वं ,
2) Inhale from the left side for a count of 16
3) hold the breath for a count of 64, and
4) breath out from the right side for a count of 32.

Now Focus the mind on the earth element. As an analogy to quickly bring your focus imagine the silvery moonlight bouncing off the rocks and trees and lighting up your body.

0) keep your attention at mooladhara the root of the spine.
1) Chant the sound yam ळं ,
2) 2) Inhale from the left side for a count of 16
3) 3) hold the breath for a count of 64, and
4) 4) breath out from the right side for a count of 32.

You may repeat this a few times say (2 or 3 times) to get the proper sequence, timing and rhythm.

एवंविधां नाडीशुद्धिं कृत्वा नाडीं विशोधयेत् । दृढो भूत्वाऽऽसनं कृत्वा प्राणायामं समाचरेत्

॥ ४५ ॥ evaṃvidhāṃ nāḍīśuddhiṃ kṛtvā nāḍīṃ viśodhayet | dṛḍho

bhūtvā"sanaṃ kṛtvā prāṇāyāmaṃ samācaret ॥ 45

5.45 These bija mantra chants practiced along with Alternate nostril breathing from left to right, help to align, create, and invigorate the grey cells of the brain.

Thus we are empowered to delve into the practice of breath regulation since our subtle being composed of nadis and chakras is now ready and functional.

सहितः सूर्यभेदश्च उज्जायी शीतली तथा । भस्त्रिका भ्रामरी मूर्च्छा केवली चाऽष्टकुम्भिकाः

॥ ४६ ॥ sahitaḥ sūryabhedaśca ujjāyī śītalī tathā | bhastrikā bhrāmarī

mūrcchā kevalī cā'ṣṭakumbhikāḥ ॥ 46

5.46 The 8 Types of breath retention or Kumbhaka which we can do during our alternate nostril breathing are
i) Sahita
ii) Suryabheda
iii) Ujjayi
iv) Shitali
v) Bhastrika
vi) Brahmari
vii) Murccha
viii) Kevali

सहितो द्विविधः प्रोक्तः सगर्भश्च निगर्भकः । सगर्भो बीजमुच्चार्य निगर्भो बीजवर्जितः ॥ ४७

sahito dvividhaḥ proktaḥ sagarbhaśca nigarbhakaḥ | sagarbho

bījamuccārya nigarbho bījavarjitaḥ ॥ 47

5.47 Sahita can be done alongside bija mantra chanting sah-garbha, or without it ni-garbhaka.

प्राणायामं सगर्भं च प्रथमं कथयामि ते । सुखाऽऽसने चोपविश्य प्राङ्मुखो वाऽप्युदङ्मुखः

। ध्यायेद्विधि रजोगुणं रक्तवर्णमवर्णकम् ॥ ४८ ॥ इडया पूरयेद्वायुं मात्रया षोडशैः सुधीः

। पूरकान्ते कुम्भकाद्ये कर्तव्यस्तूड्डियानकः ॥ ४९ ॥ सत्त्वमयं हरिं ध्यात्वा उकारं कृष्णवर्णकम् । चतुःषष्ठ्या च मात्रया कुम्भकेनैव धारयेत् । कुम्भकान्ते रेचकाद्ये कर्तव्यं च जालन्धरम् ॥ ५० ॥ तमोमयं शिवं ध्यात्वा मकारं शुक्लवर्णकम् । द्वात्रिंशन्मात्रया चैव रेचयेद्विधिना पुनः ॥ ५१ ॥ पुनः पिङ्गलयाऽऽपूर्य कुम्भकेनैव धारयेत् । इडया रेचयेत्पश्चात्तद्बीजेन क्रमेण तु ॥ ५२ ॥ prāṇāyāmaṃ sagarbhaṃ ca prathamaṃ kathayāmi te | sukhā"sane copaviśya prāṅmukho vā'pyudaṅmukhaḥ | dhyāyedvidhiṃ rajoguṇaṃ raktavarṇamavarṇakam || 48 || iḍayā pūrayedvāyuṃ mātrayā ṣoḍaśaiḥ sudhīḥ | pūrakānte kumbhakādye kartavyastūḍḍiyānakaḥ || 49 || sattvamayaṃ hariṃ dhyātvā ukāraṃ kṛṣṇavarṇakam | catuḥṣaṣṭyā ca mātrayā kumbhakenaiva dhārayet | kumbhakānte recakādye kartavyaṃ ca jālandharam || 50 || tamomayaṃ śivaṃ dhyātvā makāraṃ śuklavarṇakam | dvātriṃśanmātrayā caiva recayedvidhinā punaḥ || 51 || punaḥ piṅgalayā"pūrya kumbhakenaiva dhārayet | iḍayā recayetpaścāttadbījena krameṇa tu || 52

5.48 -52 Let's first learn the Sahita Pranayama sah-garbha alongside the chanting of the seed sound. That sound is known as the seed sound which has the requisite frequency and potential to create neurons and unlock many neural pathways.

Sit facing East or West. If your mat can only be placed along North South axis, then it is preferable to sit facing North. However irrespective of the direction, you must sit comfortably, feeling at ease.

The sukhasana posture or any posture with body relaxed yet straight is to be employed.

Contemplate on a ruddy color as a sunset full of activity - people going shopping, (buying something new as the aspect of Brahma)

birds returning home, and chant the seed sound अ (or आ or आर
as short or as long as you can).

Then we begin alternate nostril breathing. Inhale from the left
nostril for a count of 16, then apply Uddiyana bandha, then hold
the breath for a count of 64. Finally release the bandha as you
exhale through the right nostril for a count of 32.

Now inhale through the right nostril for a count of 32, apply
uddiyana bandha, hold for 64 and release the bandha as you exhale
through the left for a count of 32.

Now we chant the seed sound उ (short or long), as we
contemplate on the state of steady existence (Hari), by
remembering the magnetically attractive Krishna.

Then do one round of Nadi Shodhana Pranayam as before with
Uddiyana bandh.

Now we chant the seed sound मं , as we contemplate on the state of
continuous change (Shiva), by remembering the calm peaceful
meditative Shankara.

Then do one round of Nadi Shodhana Pranayam as before with
Uddiyana bandh.

अनुलोमविलोमेन वारं वारं च साधयेत् । पूरकान्ते कुम्भकान्तं धृतनासापुटद्वयम् ।
कनिष्ठाऽनामिकाऽङ्गुष्ठैस्तर्जनीमध्यमे विना ॥ ५३ ॥ anulomavilomena vāraṃ
vāraṃ ca sādhayet | pūrakānte kumbhakāntaṃ

dhṛtanāsāpuṭadvayam | kaniṣṭhā'nāmikā'ṅguṣṭhaistarjanīmadhyame

vinā ॥ 53

5.53 Thus we should practice Anulom Vilom or alternate nostril
breathing or Nadi Shodhana. For closing the right nostril use the
thumb, for closing the left nostril use the ring finger and little finger,

and keep the index and middle fingers free. Or you may park them on the third eye.

प्राणायामो निगर्भस्तु विना बीजेन जायते । वामजानूपरिन्यस्तवामपाणितलं भ्रमेत् । मात्रादिशतपर्यन्तं पूरकुम्भकरेचनम् ॥ ५४ ॥ prāṇāyāmo nigarbhastu vinā

bījena jāyate | vāmajānūparinyastavāmapāṇitalaṃ bhramet |

mātrādiśataparyantaṃ pūrakumbhakarecanam || 54
5.54 Now hear about the Nir-gabha Savita Anulom Vilom Pranayama.

In this simpler yet highly effective version, there is no need to visualise, nor to chant the seed sound.

The count of inhalation, retention and exhalation can be suitably varied as per individual fitness and comfort, but the ratio of 1:4:2 must be maintained.

उत्तमा विंशतिर्मात्रा षोडशी मात्रा मध्यमा । अधमा द्वादशी मात्रा प्राणायामास्त्रिधा स्मृताः

॥ ५५ ॥ uttamā viṃśatirmātrā ṣoḍaśī mātrā madhyamā | adhamā

dvādaśī mātrā prāṇāyāmāstridhā smṛtāḥ || 55
5.55 Advanced practitioners can inhale for 20 counts, the serious should inhale for 16, and the beginners can start with a count of 12 for inhalation, i.e.
Advanced Practitioners Count 20:80:40
Serious Practitioners Count 16:64:32
Beginners Count 12:48:24

अधमाज्जायते घर्मो मेरुकम्पश्च मध्यमात् । उत्तमाच्च भूमित्यागस्त्रिविधं सिद्धिलक्षणम् ॥

५६ ॥ adhamājjāyate gharmo merukampaśca madhyamāt |

uttamācca bhūmityāgastrividhaṃ siddhilakṣaṇam || 56
5.56 in the beginning if we do the Nadi Shodhana properly we shall feel warmth and integrity. As we go along for some years, we shall begin to feel quivering or vibrations. Advanced meditators shall get

a sensation of glowing light.

These indications mean that you are on the right track.

प्राणायामात्खेचरत्वं प्राणायामाद्रोगनाशनम् । प्राणायामाद्बोधयेच्छक्तिं
प्राणायामान्मनोन्मनी । आनन्दो जायते चित्ते प्राणायामी सुखी भवेत् ॥ ५७

prāṇāyāmātkhecaratvaṃ prāṇāyāmādroganāśanam |

prāṇāyāmādbodhayecchaktiṃ prāṇāyāmānmanonmanī | ānando

jāyate citte prāṇāyāmī sukhī bhavet || 57

5.57 the fruits of Pranayama are enumerated -
1) khecaratvam i.e. feeling relaxed cheerful and at ease due to
balance of senses
2) cure of illnesses if any
3) enhancement of virility
4) timely fulfilment of aspirations and desires
5) increase in intuitive faculties
The memory becomes peaceful as impressions get erased and the
practitioner derives immense success.

अथ सूर्यभेदकुम्भकः । atha sūryabhedakumbhakaḥ |

घेरण्ड उवाच । gheraṇḍa uvāca |

कथितं सहितं कुम्भं सूर्यभेदनकं शृणु । पूरयेत्सूर्यनाड्या च यथाशक्ति बहिर्मरुत् ॥ ५८
धारयेद्बहुयत्नेन कुम्भकेन जलन्धरैः । यावत्स्वेदं नखकेशाभ्यां तावत्कुर्वन्तु कुम्भकम् ॥

५९ ॥ kathitaṃ sahitaṃ kumbhaṃ sūryabhedanakaṃ śarṇu |

pūrayetsūryanāḍyā ca yathāśakti bahirmarut || 58

dhārayedbahuyatnena kumbhakena jalandharaiḥ | yāvatsvedaṃ

nakhakeśābhyāṃ tāvatkurvantu kumbhakam || 59

5.58-59 now we learn the Suryabheda kumbhaka anulom vilom
pranayama. Inhale through the right nostril long and deep, apply
jalandhar bandha, and hold the breath for a comfortable period,
then exhale slowly through the left.

Repeat this sequence of inhalation through right, applying jalandhar bandha, holding the breath and releasing through the left.

Prana Vayu and Upaprana Vayu

प्राणोपानः समानश्चोदानव्यानौ तथैव च । नागः कूर्मश्च कृकरो देवदत्तो धनञ्जयः ॥ ६०

prāṇo'pānaḥ samānaścodānavyānau tathaiva ca | nāgaḥ kūrmaśca

kṛkaro devadatto dhanañjayaḥ || 60

5.60 hear the 5 types of prana airs and 5 types of upa-prana airs.
1. Prana for respiratory
2. Apana for excretory
3. Samana for circulatory
4. Udana for
5. Vyana
The 5 upa-prana vayus are
1. Naga
2. Kurma
3. Krikara
4. Devdutta
5. Dhananjaya

हृदि प्राणो वहेन्नित्यमपानो गुदमण्डले । समानो नाभिदेशे तु उदानः कण्ठमध्यगः ॥ ६१

hṛdi prāṇo vahennityamapāno gudamaṇḍale | samāno nābhideśe tu

udānaḥ kaṇṭhamadhyagaḥ || 61

5.61 The prana vayu moves in the center of the chest, the apana in the abdomen, samana in the navel, udana at the throat, and vyana pervades the whole body.

The 5 principal airs prana etc are related to the core anatomical systems. The 5 subsidiary airs naga etc are related to the peripheral anatomical systems.

व्यानो व्याप्य शरीरे तु प्रधानाः पञ्च वायवः । प्राणाद्याः पञ्च विख्याता नागाद्याः पञ्च

वायवः ॥ ६२ ॥ vyāno vyāpya śarīre tu pradhānāḥ pañca vāyavaḥ |

prāṇādyāḥ pañca vikhyātā nāgādyāḥ pañca vāyavaḥ ॥ 62

5.62 We now see the functions of the upa-prana vayus

1) naga drives erotic erection or arousal

2) kurma makes the eyelids droop or close and open

3) krikara causes sneezing

4) devaduta controls yawning

5) Dhananjaya is responsible for rigor mortis and post death functions

तेषामपि च पञ्चानां स्थानानि च वदाम्यहम् । उद्गारे नाग आख्यातः कूर्मस्तून्मीलने स्मृतः ॥ ६३ ॥ कृकरः क्षुत्कृते ज्ञेयो देवदत्तो विजृम्भणे । न जहाति मृते क्वाऽपि सर्वव्यापी धनञ्जयः ॥ ६४ ॥ नागो गृह्णाति चैतन्यं कूर्मश्चैव निमेषणम् । क्षुत्तृषं कृकरश्चैव जृम्भणं चतुर्थेन तु । भवेद्धनञ्जयाच्छब्दं क्षणमात्रं न निःसरेत् चित्तं धनञ्जयः शब्दं लक्षमात्रं न विस्मरेत् ॥ ६५ ॥ teṣāmapi ca pañcānāṃ sthānāni ca vadāmyaham |

udgāre nāga ākhyātaḥ kūrmastūnmīlane smṛtaḥ ॥ 63 ॥ kṛkaraḥ

kṣutkṛte jñeyo devadatto vijṛmbhaṇe | na jahāti mṛte kvā'pi

sarvavyāpī dhanañjayaḥ ॥ 64 ॥ nāgo gṛhṇāti caitanyaṃ

kūrmaścaiva nimeṣaṇam | kṣuttṛṣaṃ kṛkaraścaiva jṛmbhaṇaṃ

caturthena tu | bhaveddhanañjayācchabdaṃ kṣaṇamātraṃ na

niḥsaret cittaṃ dhanañjayaḥ śabdaṃ lakṣamātraṃ na vismaret ॥ 65

5.63-65 more about upa-prana vayus

1) naga also governs virility and vitality

2) kurma plays a role in health of eye muscles and retina

3) kirkira causes hunger pangs or parched throat

4) devadutta gives rise to day dreams

5) Dhananjaya helps make sounds intelligible and makes our audiometry function

अथ सूर्यभेदकः कुम्भकः । atha sūryabhedakaḥ kumbhakaḥ |

सर्वे ते सूर्यसम्भिन्ना नाभिमूलात्समुद्धरेत् । इडया रेचयेत्पश्चाद्धैर्येणाऽखण्डवेगतः ॥ ६६

पुनः सूर्येण चाऽऽकृष्य कुम्भयित्वा यथाविधि । रेचयित्वा साधयेत्तु क्रमेण च पुनः पुनः ॥

६७ ॥ sarve te sūryasambhinnā nābhimūlātsamuddharet | iḍayā

recayetpaścāddhairyeṇā'khaṇḍavegataḥ ॥ 66

punaḥ sūryeṇa cā'kṛṣya kumbhayitvā yathāvidhi | recayitvā

sādhayettu krameṇa ca punaḥ punaḥ ॥ 67
5.66-67 Suryabheda Pranayama alongside jalandhar bandha and kumbhaka regulates the functioning of upa-prana vayus.

For Suryabheda always inhale through right nostril and exhale through left nostril. Continue it for few minutes and then relax, being still and silent for couple of minutes as the effects of Pranayama get established in the body.

कुम्भकः सूर्यभेदस्तु जरामृत्युविनाशकः । बोधयेत्कुण्डलीं शक्ति देहानलं विवर्धयेत् ।
इति ते कथितं चण्ड सूर्यभेदनमुत्तमम् ॥ ६८ ॥ kumbhakaḥ sūryabhedastu

jarāmṛtyuvināśakaḥ | bodhayetkuṇḍalīṃ śaktiṃ dehānalaṃ

vivardhayet | iti te kathitaṃ caṇḍa sūryabhedanamuttamam ॥ 68
5.68 Its regular practice keeps the body flexible and fit well into ripe old age. The upa-prana vayus control a number of secondary functions, which are crucial in general health and enthusiasm, imagination and planning, and alertness of senses.

Ujjayi Breath अथ उज्जायी कुम्भकः ।

नासाभ्यां वायुमाकृष्य मुखमध्ये च धारयेत् । हृद्गलाभ्यां समाकृष्य वायुं वक्रे च धारयेत् ॥
६९ ॥ मुखं प्रफुल्लं संरक्ष्य कुर्याज्जालन्धरं ततः । आशक्ति कुम्भकं कृत्वा धारयेदविरोधतः

॥ ७० ॥ nāsābhyāṃ vāyumākṛṣya mukhamadhye ca dhārayet |

hṛdgalābhyāṃ samākṛṣya vāyuṃ vaktre ca dhārayet ॥ 69

mukhaṃ praphullaṃ saṃrakṣya kuryājjālandharaṃ tataḥ | āśakti

kumbhakaṃ kṛtvā dhārayedavirodhataḥ ॥ 70

5.69-70 we now learn Ujjayi Kumbhaka Pranayama. Inhale deeply drawing the air so that it massages the throat muscles, and the sound of friction is heard clearly.

Then hold the breath as long as is comfortable. Then release again with the breath massaging the throat area and the friction sound is clearly audible.

After exhalation, apply Jalandhar bandha. Release the bandha slowly and with full concentration.

Then repeat the process
1) ujjayi breath in
2) kumbhaka
3) ujjayi breath out
4) jalandhar bandha

Continue these cycles for a few minutes, and then become silent and still for a couple of minutes, so that the effects of the Pranayama get established.

Note that it will take at least 40 days for the inhalations to become slow and deep, for the kumbhaka release to become jerk free, and for the effects of the Pranayama to be distinctly noticeable in general health and enthusiasm levels. You will also see that your mind has become more open, accepting, and unpolarised.

उज्जायीकुम्भकं कृत्वा सर्वकार्याणि साधयेत् । न भवेत्कफरोगश्च क्रूरवायुरजीर्णकम् ॥ ७१
आमवातः क्षयः कासो ज्वरप्लीहा न विद्यते । जरामृत्युविनाशाय चोज्जायीं साधयेन्नरः ॥ ७२

ujjāyīkumbhakaṃ kṛtvā sarvakāryāṇi sādhayet I na

bhavetkapharogaśca krūravāyurajīrṇakam II 71

āmavātaḥ kṣayaḥ kāso jvaraplīhā na vidyate I jarāmṛtyuvināśāya

cojjāyīṃ sādhayennaraḥ I naśyanti sakalā rogāḥ sādhanādasya

niścitam II 72

5.71-72 Ujjayi breathing helps to reduce the sensory excitements, while the added kumbhaka dismantles those neural networks where such excitements keep getting stored and the added jalandhar bandha prevents throat and lung infections.

Thus the Ujjayi pranayama keeps the brain fit and functional well into old age, preventing nervous disorders. Also since throat and lung fitness improve, the breath capacity increases significantly, and hence the effects become long-lasting.

अथ शीतलीकुम्भकः । atha śītalīkumbhakaḥ ।

जिह्वया वायुमाकृष्य उदरे पूरयेच्छनैः । क्षणं च कुम्भकं कृत्वा नासाभ्यां रेचयेत्पुनः ॥ ७३

jihvayā vāyumākṛṣya udare pūrayecchanaiḥ । kṣaṇaṃ ca kumbhakam

kṛtvā nāsābhyāṃ recayetpunah ॥ 73

5.73 Hear about Sitali Kumbhaka Pranayama.
1) take the tongue out and make a tube puckering the mouth
2) suck in air through the tongue tube
3) hold the breath for few seconds
4) exhale slowly through the nose.

सर्वदा साधयेद्योगी शीतलीकुम्भकं शुभम् । अजीर्णं कफपित्तं च नैव तस्य प्रजायते ॥ ७४

sarvadā sādhayedyogī śītalīkumbhakaṃ śubham । ajīrṇaṃ

kaphapittaṃ ca naiva tasya prajāyate ॥ 74

5.74 Sitali must be practiced only in warm weather, or when it is not chilly.

Avoid it when you have a cold.

It provides cooling sensation in the brain, and soothes the tired nerves.

Bhastrika अथ भस्त्रिकाकुम्भकः ।

भस्त्रैव लोहकाराणां यथाक्रमेण सम्भ्रमेत् । तथा वायुं च नासाभ्यामुभाभ्यां चालयेच्छनैः

॥ ७५ ॥ bhastraiva lohakārāṇāṃ yathākrameṇa sambhramet | tathā

vāyuṃ ca nāsābhyāmubhābhyāṃ cālayecchanaiḥ ॥ 75

5.75 Bhastrika Pranayama is akin to the working of the bellows of an iron Smith or using a bicycle pump to fill air in the tyre.

We breath in applying measurable force expanding the stomach, then suddenly expel all the air in a jerk.

Bhastrika produces a loud unpleasant sound, and should be avoided in public places or when a function is going on.

एवं विंशतिवारं च कृत्वा कुर्याच्च कुम्भकम् । तदन्ते चालयेद्वायुं पूर्वोक्तं च यथाविधि ॥ ७६
त्रिवारं साधयेदेनं भस्त्रिकाकुम्भकं सुधीः । न च रोगो न च क्लेश आरोग्यं च दिने दिने ॥

७७ ॥ evaṃ vimśativāraṃ ca kṛtvā kuryācca kumbhakam | tadante

cālayedvāyuṃ pūrvoktaṃ ca yathāvidhi ॥ 76

trivāraṃ sādhayedenam bhastrikākumbhakaṃ sudhīḥ | na ca rogo na

ca kleśa ārogyaṃ ca dine dine ॥ 77

5.76-77 Bhastrika must be done for a count of 20 in one round. Then Kumbhaka.

Repeat 3 such rounds.

Bhastrika will heal the tissues. It works on the cellular level and expels all the stale air from our organs and joints.

Without our knowing, air from many days or even months keeps rotting in our innards, without finding any release. Even many alveoli in the lungs never get to experience fresh air. Bhastrika is one such easily doable no cost at home routine we all can implement in our daily routine.

It speeds up the processes that occur during sleep, viz repair and maintenance of the anatomy. It ensures fresh oxygen to some parts of the body which have not been attended to in a long time due to our faulty posture or incorrect lifestyle.

Brahmari or OM अथ भ्रामरीकुम्भकः ।

अर्धरात्रे गते योगी जन्तूनां शब्दवर्जिते । कर्णौ पिधाय हस्ताभ्यां कुर्यात्पूरककुम्भकम् ॥ ७८ ॥ शृणुयाद्दक्षिणे कर्णे नादमन्तर्गतं शुभम् । प्रथमं जिंजीनादं च वंशीनादं ततः परम् ॥ ७९ ॥ मेघजर्जरभ्रामरी घण्टाकांस्यं ततः परम् । तुरीभेरीमृदङ्गादिनिनादानकदुन्दुभिः ॥ ८० ॥ ardharātre gate yogī jantūnāṃ śabdavarjite | karṇau pidhāya

hastābhyāṃ kuryātpūrakakumbhakam ॥ 78 ॥ śarṇuyāddakṣiṇe

karṇe nādamantargataṃ śubham | prathamaṃ jiṃjīnādaṃ ca

vaṃśīnādaṃ tataḥ param ॥ 79 ॥ meghajarjarabhrāmarī

ghaṇṭākāṃsyam tataḥ param |

turībherīmṛdaṅgādininādānakadundubhiḥ ॥ 80
5.78 -80 Brahmari Kumbhaka Pranayama is now told.
1) close you eyes and
2) inhale slowly through the nose
3) hold the breath for a few seconds
4) now shut both ears using the thumbs and exhale slowly, while making a humming bee sound
5) repeat this Brahmari a few times
6) then sit still and silent. If you like you may lie down and rest.
7) only then the effects of Brahmari get internalized.

If we can practice Brahmari early morning when nature is silent and there is no traffic noise, then we can hear some magnified internal body sounds. We may hear the sound of crickets and buzzing insects. We may hear the sound of a string instrument, the thunder of a passing aeroplane. Or even the sounds of various drums and musical instruments.

These are the sounds of the body factory which normally we are unaware of.

एवं नानाविधो नादो जायते नित्यमभ्यसात् । अनाहतस्य शब्दस्य तस्य शब्दस्य यो ध्वनिः ॥ ८१ ॥ ध्वनेरन्तर्गतं ज्योतिज्योतिरन्तर्गतं मनः । तन्मनो विलयं याति तद्विष्णोः परमं पदम् । एवं भ्रामरीसंसिद्धिः समाधिसिद्धिमाप्नुयात् ॥ ८२

evaṃ nānāvidho nādo jāyate nityamabhyasāt | anāhatasya śabdasya tasya śabdasya yo dhvaniḥ ‖ 81 ‖ dhvanerantargataṃ jyotirjyotirantargataṃ manaḥ | tanmano vilayaṃ yāti tadviṣṇoḥ paramaṃ padam | evaṃ bhrāmarīsaṃsiddhiḥ samādhisiddhimāpnuyāt ‖ 82

5.81-82 It takes a couple of years for the Brahmari Kumbhaka Practice to be well integrated. Only then are these faint sounds cognized.

Also we can notice if there is resonance or dissonance, depending upon our state of mind and condition of the heart.

After many years of diligent practice, one may become aware of the sound of the soul ... the sound that is produced without any cause, without the vibration from any physical, anatomical or nervous activity.

This sound known as the anhat naad unstruck sound, is heard only in deep states of meditation. It is experienced rarely, it is very healing, and sometimes a soft luminous glow is also noticed.

Brahmari is highly recommended for satvik or rajasic temperaments. However those having depression should avoid it completely.

Brahmari fills the mind with bliss and lends success in ventures to the practitioner.

अथ मूर्च्छाकुम्भकः । atha mūrcchākumbhakaḥ |

सुखेन कुम्भकं कृत्वा मनश्च भ्रुवोरन्तरम् । सन्त्यज्य विषयान्सर्वान्मनोमूर्च्छा सुखप्रदा ।
आत्मनि मनसो योगादानन्दो जायते ध्रुवम् ॥ ८३

sukhena kumbhakaṃ kṛtvā manaśca bhruvorantaram | santyajya

viṣayānsarvānmanomūrcchā sukhapradā | ātmani manaso

yogādānando jāyate dhruvam ‖ 83
5.83 Murchha Pranayama or Dazed technique.
1) inhale deeply through the nose
2) apply kumbhaka for as long as comfortable
3) as you release the breath slowly, focus your eyes to stare at your eyebrows
4) within few seconds you shall feel a bit dazed as if fainting
5) let go relax and be still and silent for a while

We do this only once. We do not do it daily, only rarely.

SoHam Kriya

हङ्कारेण बहिर्याति सःकारेण विशेत्पुनः । षट्शतानि दिवारात्रौ सहस्राण्येकविंशतिः ।
अजपां नाम गायत्री जीवो जपति सर्वदा ॥ ८४ ॥ haṅkāreṇa bahiryāti

saḥkāreṇa viśetpunaḥ | ṣaṭśatāni divārātrau sahasrāṇyekaviṃśatiḥ |

ajapāṃ nāma gāyatrīṃ jīvo japati sarvadā ‖ 84
5.84 (Kevali Kumbhaka Pranayama or Rhythmic Breathing)
As the breath goes out it makes the sound हम् and as it comes in, it

makes the sound सः , written together it is सः अहम् or सोऽहम् by

the Sanskrit grammar sandhi rules. In English सोऽहम् is

transliterated as Soham.

In a 24-hour day, there is a count of 600 and 21 thousand such respirations. This unhindered continuous respiration is directly governed by an invisible force.

The Soham breath is the breath to be done consciously every

single day. We can learn it properly by attending the Art of Living Happiness course.

It is called Sudarshan Kriya and it was first cognized and revealed to the world by Gurudev Sri Sri Ravi Shankar.

मूलाधारे यथा हंसस्तथा हि हृदि पङ्कजे । तथा नासापुटद्वन्द्वे त्रिभिर्हंससमागमः ॥ ८५

mūlā"dhāre yathā haṃsastathā hi hṛdi paṅkaje | tathā

nāsāpuṭadvandve tribhirhaṃsasamāgamaḥ ‖ 85

5.85 There are three key areas of our spine which get superbly nourished and attended to by the Soham breath. The base of the spine known as the Mooladhara Chakra or all organs of our pelvic waist, the center of the chest known as the Anahata Chakra which defines and coordinates the major organs like the lungs and heart, and the Ajna chakra that helps in all decision making.

षण्णवत्यङ्गुलीमानं शरीरं कर्मरूपकम् । देहाद्बहिर्गतो वायुः स्वभावाद्द्वादशाङ्गुलिः ॥ ८६

गायने षोडशाङ्गुल्यो भोजने विंशतिस्तथा । चतुर्विंशाङ्गुलिः पन्थे निद्रायां त्रिंशदङ्गुलिः ।

मैथुने षड्त्रिंशदुक्तं व्यायामे च ततोऽधिकम् ॥ ८७

ṣaṇṇavatyaṅgulīmānaṃ śarīraṃ karmarūpakam | dehādbahirgato

vāyuḥ svabhāvāddvādaśāṅguliḥ ‖ 86

gāyane ṣoḍaśāṅgulyo bhojane viṃśatistathā | caturviṃśāṅguliḥ

panthe nidrāyāṃ triṃśadaṅguliḥ | maithune ṣaṭṭriṃśaduktaṃ

vyāyāme ca tato'dhikam ‖ 87

5.86-87 our aural body extends six inches in all directions. The tempo of our breath varies with our activity,
-Sitting = 12 finger digits
-singing = 16 finger digits
-eating = 20
-walking = 24
-sleeping = 30
-romantic excitement = 36
-ploughing and other physical chores = much more

स्वभावेऽस्य गतेर्न्यूने परमायुः प्रवर्धते । आयुःक्षयोऽधिके प्रोक्तो मारुते चाऽन्तराद्गते ॥

८८ ॥ svabhāve'sya gaternyūne paramāyuḥ pravardhate |

āyuḥkṣayo'dhike prokto mārute cā'ntarādgate ॥ 88

5.88 by minimising the strain of breathing from exhaustion, the life force increases manifold, whereas by breathing in pain whether physical or mental, the prana becomes reduced.

One must strive to maximize our prana by doing conscious Soham breathing daily.

तस्मात्प्राणे स्थिते देहे मरणं नैव जायते । वायुना घटसम्बन्धे भवेत्केवलकुम्भकम् ॥ ८९

tasmātprāṇe sthite dehe maraṇaṃ naiva jāyate | vāyunā

ghaṭasambandhe bhavetkevalakumbhakam ॥ 89

5.89 this coordinated breath is known as Keval Kumbhaka, as it harmonises all aspects of the being and makes old age smooth and death painless.

यावज्जीवं जपेन्मन्त्रमजपासङ्ख्यकेवलम् सङ्ख्या द्विगुणा । अद्यावधि धृतं सङ्ख्याविभ्रमं केवलीकृते ॥ ९० ॥ अत एव हि कर्तव्यः केवलीकुम्भको नरैः । केवली चाऽजपासङ्ख्या द्विगुणा च मनोन्मनी ॥ ९१

yāvajjīvaṃ japenmantramajapāsaṅkhyakevalam saṅkhyā dviguṇā |

adyāvadhi dhṛtaṃ saṅkhyāvibhramam kevalīkṛte ॥ 90

ata eva hi kartavyaḥ kevalīkumbhako naraiḥ | kevalī cā'japāsaṅkhyā

dviguṇā ca manonmanī ॥ 91

5.90-91 we saw earlier that normal respirations are 15 per minute or 150 in ten minutes. By doubling this, i.e. doing 300 respirations in ten minutes as in Sudarshan Kriya, once a day, we can achieve long term
General fitness and purity in heart. This kriya is known as Manonmani, the way to win over the mind. Guruji calls it Sudarshan Kriya.

In this Kriya, there is only the rhythmic breathing, no specific posture, nor any chanting, nor any visualisation. This is known as the Yogic way, or knowing how to live balanced and integrated.

नासाभ्यां वायुमाकृष्य केवलं कुम्भकं चरेत् । एकादिकचतुःषष्टिं धारयेत्प्रथमे दिने ॥ ९२

nāsābhyāṃ vāyumākṛṣya kevalaṃ kumbhakaṃ caret |

ekādikacatuḥṣaṣṭiṃ dhārayetprathame dine ‖ 92

5.92 In the rhythmic breathing Kevali Kumbhaka process, air is inhaled from both the nostrils, not from the mouth.

Prior to it, (sixty-four) eight eight rounds of deep breathing may be done.

केवलीमष्टधा कुर्याद्यामे यामे दिने दिने । अथवा पञ्चधा कुर्याद्यथा तत्कथयामि ते ॥ ९३
प्रातर्मध्याह्नसायाह्ने मध्ये रात्रिचतुर्थके । त्रिसन्ध्यमथवा कुर्यात्सममाने दिने दिने ॥ ९४

kevalīmaṣṭadhā kuryādyāme yāme dine dine | athavā pañcadhā

kuryādyathā tatkathayāmi te ‖ 93

prātarmadhyāhnasāyāhne madhye rātricaturthake |

trisandhyamathavā kuryātsamamāne dine dine ‖ 94

5.93-94 Long Deep breath for a count of eight rounds is beneficial.

There are five components to the kriya, including ujjayi breath, bhastrika, om chanting, rhythmic breathing, and lying down or becoming still and silent.

For maximum results, we can do the rhythmic breathing kriya at dawn, or noon, or dusk. At these hours the nature is especially benevolent.

पञ्चवारं दिने वृद्धिविरेकं च दिने तथा । अजपापरिमाणं च यावत्सिद्धिः प्रजायते ॥ ९५

pañcavāraṃ dine vṛddhirvāraikaṃ ca dine tathā | ajapāparimāṇaṃ ca yāvatsiddhiḥ prajāyate || 95

5.95 Best to do all five components of the process.
He who practices this form of Pranayama attains to true yoga.

प्राणायामं केवलीं च तदा वदति योगवित् । केवलीकुम्भके सिद्धे किं न सिध्यति भूतले॥९६

prāṇāyāmaṃ kevalīṃ ca tadā vadati yogavit | kevalīkumbhake siddhe kiṃ na sidhyati bhūtale || 96

5.96 One must keep up the practice of rhythmic breathing until it becomes second nature.

What type of success be evaded, what target be unattainable, for the one who does this kriya with commitment, regularity and cheerfulness?

|| इति श्रीघेरण्डसंहितायां घेरण्डचण्डसंवादे घटस्थयोगप्रकरणे प्राणायामप्रयोगो नाम पञ्चमोपदेशः || iti śrīgheraṇḍasaṃhitāyāṃ gheraṇḍacaṇḍasaṃvāde ghaṭasthayogaprakaraṇe prāṇāyāmaprayogo nāma pañcamopadeśaḥ || Here ends the most important Teaching section of this dialogue.

6 Meditation - Dhyana ध्यानयोगो नाम षष्ठोपदेशः

घेरण्ड उवाच । gheraṇḍa uvāca । स्थूलं ज्योतिस्तथा सूक्ष्मं ध्यानस्य त्रिविधं विदुः ।
स्थूलं मूर्तिमयं प्रोक्तं ज्योतिस्तेजोमयं तथा । सूक्ष्मं बिन्दुमयं ब्रह्म कुण्डलीपरदेवता ॥ १

sthūlaṃ jyotistathā sūkṣmaṃ dhyānasya trividhaṃ viduḥ |

sthūlaṃ mūrtimayaṃ proktaṃ jyotistejomayaṃ tathā |

sūkṣmaṃ bindumayaṃ brahma kuṇḍalīparadevatā ॥ 1

6.1 gross, luminous and subtle, these are the three kinds of
meditative contemplation, known as dhyana.

In gross meditation we contemplate on our favorite deity
In luminous meditation we remember a flame or glow.
That is called subtle meditation when just a tiny point is visualised.

In all cases our dormant energy gets activated and we move towards
the plane of freedom from misery.

अथ स्थूलध्यानम् । atha sthūladhyānam |
स्वकीयहृदये ध्यायेत्सुधासागरमुत्तमम् । तन्मध्ये रत्नद्वीपं तु सुरत्नवालुकामयम् ॥ २

svakīyahṛdaye dhyāyetsudhāsāgaramuttamam |

tanmadhye ratnadvīpaṃ tu suratnavālukāmayam ॥ 2

6.2 We first make ourselves immersed in contemplating what is very
attractive to the senses. Begin by thinking of diamonds and rubies
and acknowledge the sensations that arise.

चतुर्दिक्षु नीपतरुं बहुपुष्पसमन्वितम् । नीपोपवनसङ्कुलैर्वेष्टितं परिखा इव ॥ ३

caturdikṣu nīpataruṃ bahupuṣpasamanvitam |

nīpopavanasaṅkulairveṣṭitaṃ parikhā iva ॥ 3

मालतीमल्लिकाजातीकेसरैश्चम्पकैस्तथा । पारिजातैः स्थलपद्मैर्गन्धामोदितदिङ्मुखैः ॥ ४

mālatīmallikājātīkesaraiścampakaistathā |

pārijātaiḥ sthalapadmairgandhāmoditadiṅmukhaiḥ ॥ 4

6.3-4 Then think of fragrant sweet-smelling flowers.

तन्मध्ये संस्मरेद्योगी कल्पवृक्षं मनोहरम् । चतुःशाखाचतुर्वेदं नित्यपुष्पफलान्वितम् ॥ ५

tanmadhye saṃsmaredyogī kalpavṛkṣaṃ manoharam |

catuḥśākhācaturvedaṃ nityapuṣpaphalānvitam ॥ 5

6.5 Then of seeing the body of high knowledge being accessed and grasped in a loving environment.

भ्रमराः कोकिलास्तत्र गुञ्जन्ति निगदन्ति च । ध्यायेत्तत्र स्थिरो भूत्वा महामाणिक्यमण्डपम्

॥ ६ ॥ bhramarāḥ kokilāstatra guñjanti nigadanti ca | dhyāyettatra

sthiro bhūtvā mahāmāṇikyamaṇḍapam ॥ 6

6.6 Then the sounds of great music and orchestra.

तन्मध्ये तु स्मरेद्योगी पर्यङ्कं सुमनोहरम् । तत्रेष्टदेवतां ध्यायेद्यद्ध्यानं गुरुभाषितम् ॥ ७

tanmadhye tu smaredyogī paryaṅkaṃ sumanoharam |

tatreṣṭadevatāṃ dhyāyedyaddhyānaṃ gurubhāṣitam ॥ 7

6.7 Finally get absorbed in visualising your chosen ideal and aim, as taught to you by your Master.

यस्य देवस्य यद्रूपं यथा भूषणवाहनम् । तद्रूपं ध्यायते नित्यं स्थूलध्यानमिदं विदुः ॥ ८

yasya devasya yadrūpaṃ yathā bhūṣaṇavāhanam | tadrūpaṃ

dhyāyate nityaṃ sthūladhyānamidaṃ viduḥ ॥ 8

6.8 When one merges with such imaginings, the mind becomes withdrawn and settles down. This is a gross yet highly effective method of activating our dormant life force.

सहस्रारे महापद्मे कर्णिकायां विचिन्तयेत् । विलग्नसहितं पद्मं द्वादशैर्दलसंयुतम् ॥ ९

sahasrāre mahāpadme karṇikāyāṃ vicintayet |

vilagnasahitaṃ padmaṃ dvādaśairdalasaṃyutam ॥ 9

शुक्लवर्णं महातेजो द्वादशैर्बीजभाषितम् । हसक्षमलवरयुं हसखफ्रें यथाक्रमम् ॥ १०

śuklavarṇaṃ mahātejo dvādaśairbījabhāṣitam |

hasakṣamalavarayuṃ hasakhaphreṃ yathākramam || 10

तन्मध्ये कर्णिकायां तु अकथादिरेखात्रयम् । हळक्षकोणसंयुक्तं प्रणवं तत्र वर्तते ॥ ११

tanmadhye karṇikāyāṃ tu akathādirekhātrayam |

halakṣakoṇasaṃyuktaṃ praṇavaṃ tatra vartate || 11

6.9 – 11 Let the seeker contemplate on a thousand petalled lotus, and bring his attention to the center of his brain. Now let him visualize a snow white twelve petalled lotus, while taking his awareness deep inside the brain to the hypothalamus and amegdala. Let him imagine the glowing petals having the 12 seed letters - ह स क्ष मम ल व र युं ह स ख फ्रें । And touching the circumference of this lotus an equilateral triangle is formed by three lines named अ ख थ with the angles named ह ळ क्ष ।

In the exact center of this radiant triangle is the sacred sound Om.

Guruji, two Swans and Paduka

नादबिन्दुमयं पीठं ध्यायेत्तत्र मनोहरम् । तत्रोपरि हंसयुग्मं पादुका तत्र वर्तते ॥ १२

nādabindumayaṃ pīṭhaṃ dhyāyettatra manoharam |

tatropari haṃsayugmaṃ pādukā tatra vartate || 12

6.12 in such a divine place filled with the sacred sound, let him fix his thought on a fine point of light.

Soon he becomes aware of two milk-white Swans, and the holy feet of his Guru.

ध्यायेत्तत्र गुरुं देवं द्विभुजं च त्रिलोचनम् । श्वेताम्बरधरं देवं शुक्लगन्धानुलेपनम् ॥ १३

dhyāyettatra gurum devaṃ dvibhujaṃ ca trilocanam |

śvetāmbaradharam devaṃ śuklagandhānulepanam || 13

6.13 The Guru is dressed in spotless white, the graceful hands and large piercing eyes, and third eye also evident.

शुक्लपुष्पमयं माल्यं रक्तशक्तिसमन्वितम् । एवंविधगुरुध्यानात्स्थूलध्यानं प्रसिध्यति ॥ १४

śuklapuṣpamayaṃ mālyaṃ raktaśaktisamanvitam |

evaṃvidhagurudhyānātsthūladhyānaṃ prasidhyati || 14

6.14 Guruji sports a jasmine garland, his forehead is adorned with sandalwood paste, and a powerful energy surrounds him.

When this apparition manifests know that you have succeeded in the gross meditation, and your energy centers have been activated.

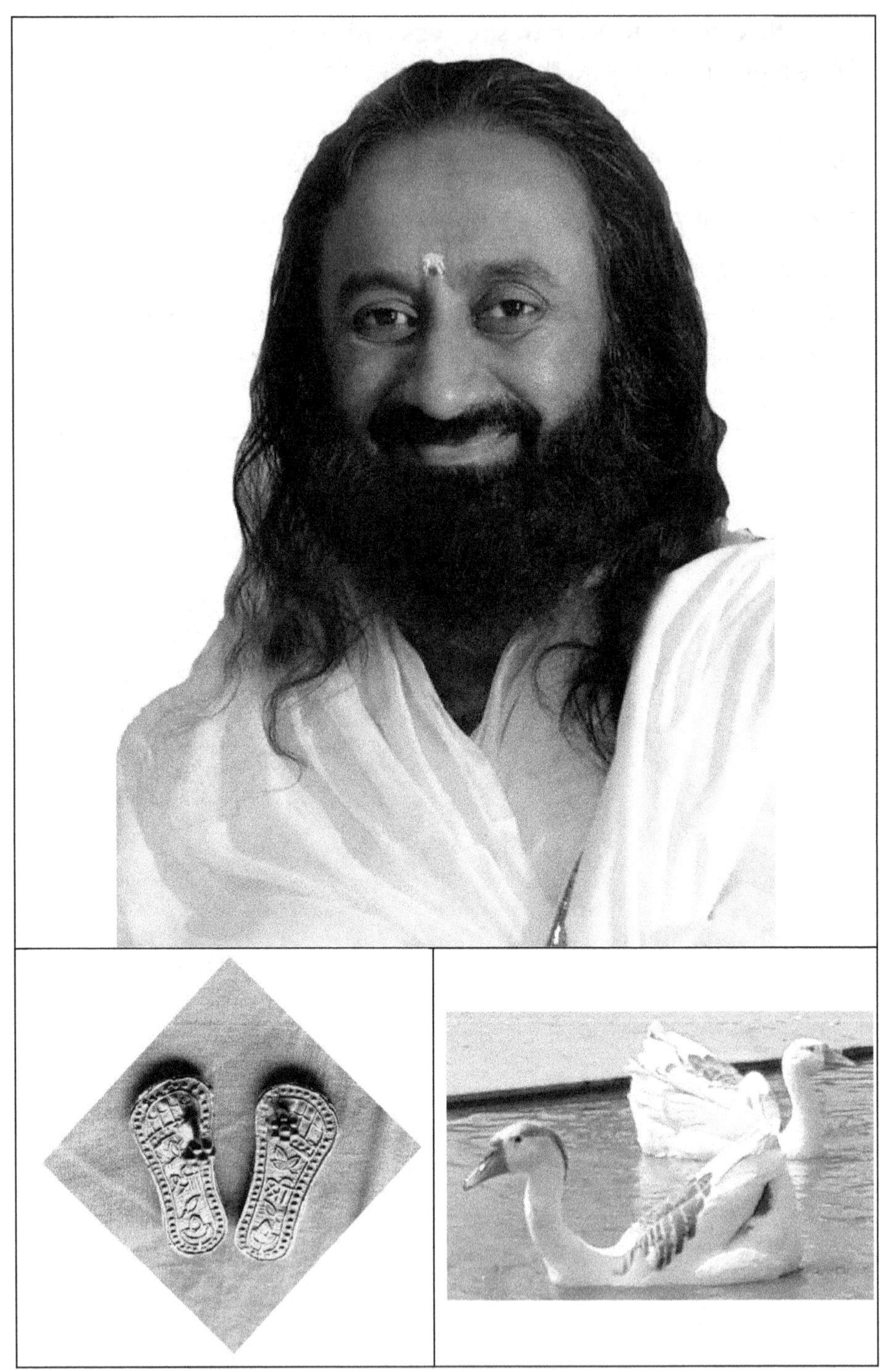

अथ ज्योतिर्ध्यानम् । atha jyotirdhyānam । घेरण्ड उवाच । gheraṇḍa uvāca ।
कथितं स्थूलध्यानं तु तेजोध्यानं शृणुष्व मे । यद्ध्यानेन योगसिद्धिरात्मप्रत्यक्षमेव च ॥ १५

kathitaṃ sthūladhyānaṃ tu tejodhyānaṃ śarṇuṣva me ।

yaddhyānena yogasiddhirātmapratyakṣameva ca ॥ 15

6.15 Hear now a method of luminous meditation. Its soft glow shall transport you to the plane of Brahman, where there is no sorrow, and once having gotten such an experience, your memory shall never again be blemished.

मूलाऽऽधारे कुण्डलिनी भुजगाकाररूपिणी । जीवाऽऽत्मा तिष्ठति तत्र प्रदीपकलिकाकृतिः । ध्यायेत्तेजोमयं ब्रह्म तेजोध्यानं परात्परम् ॥ १६ ॥ jīvā"tmā tiṣṭhati tatra

pradīpakalikākṛtiḥ । dhyāyettejomayaṃ brahma tejodhyānaṃ

parātparam ॥ 16

6.16 In the mooladhara at the base of the spine resides the dormant kundalini shakti, or infinite life force. It is lying like a dormant serpent, limpless, coiled like a rope.

The soul resides in the cave of one's heart, contemplate on a loving thought entering the luminous soul.

This makes us touch base with Brahman, the omnipotent super consciousness, and one is immediately healed.

नाभिमूले स्थितं सूर्यमण्डलं वह्निसंयुतम् । ध्यायेत्तेजो महद्व्याप्तं तेजोध्यानं तदेव हि ॥ १७

nābhimūle sthitaṃ sūryamaṇḍalaṃ vahnisaṃyutam ।

dhyāyettejo mahadvyāptaṃ tejodhyānaṃ tadeva hi ॥ 17

6.17 One can also focus on a tiny luminous point in the manipura chakra or solar plexus, and similarly attain oneness with Brahman.

भ्रुवोर्मध्ये मनोर्ध्वे च यत्तेजः प्रणवाऽऽत्मकम् । ध्यायेज्ज्वालाऽऽवलीयुक्तं तेजोध्यानं तदेव हि ॥ १८ ॥ bhruvormadhye manordhve ca yattejaḥ praṇavā"tmakam

dhyāyejjvālā''valīyuktaṃ tejodhyānaṃ tadeva hi ‖ 18
6.18 Or one may focus on a tiny luminous point on one's third eye in
between the eyebrows, and similarly attain oneness with Brahman.

अथ सूक्ष्मध्यानम् । atha sūkṣmadhyānam । घेरण्ड उवाच। gheraṇḍa uvāca ।

तेजोध्यानं श्रुतं चण्ड सूक्ष्मध्यानं शृणुष्व मे । बहुभाग्यवशाद्यस्य कुण्डली जाग्रती भवेत्

‖ १९ ‖ tejodhyānaṃ śrutaṃ caṇḍa sūkṣmadhyānaṃ śarṇuṣva me ।

bahubhāgyavaśādyasya kuṇḍalī jāgratī bhavet ‖ 19
6.19 O pleasant one! You have learnt the luminous meditation, now
we proceed with the subtle meditation.

This is the path of good fortune. This meditation is had by Guru
Grace and lots of Tapas. It is the proper awakening of the dormant
energy we have all been gifted with in this human nervous system.

आत्मना सह योगेन नेत्ररन्ध्राद्विनिर्गता । विहरेद्राजमार्गे च चञ्चलत्वान्न दृश्यते ‖ २०

ātmanā saha yogena netrarandhrādvinirgatā ।

viharedrājamārge ca cañcalatvānna dṛśyate ‖ 20
6.20 the soul moves out of the two eyes when happy and
contented. The proper flow of satvik energy within the nervous
system alone can cause such an exit.

This may not be apparent nor easily detected, since the soul's
movements are beyond the senses and intellect.

शाम्भवीमुद्रया योगी ध्यानयोगेन सिध्यति ।सूक्ष्मध्यानमिदं गोप्यं देवानामपि दुर्लभम्‖२१

śāmbhavīmudrayā yogī dhyānayogena sidhyati ।

sūkṣmadhyānamidaṃ gopyaṃ devānāmapi durlabham ‖ 21
6 21 one of the techniques to help the soul's movement is the
Shambhavi mudra, as it ensures proper flow of the kundalini
current.

However these techniques are rarely taught, and the Guru chooses the few brilliant disciples who have maintained a satvik respectful and helpful attitude over many years.

स्थूलध्यानाच्छतगुणं तेजोध्यानं प्रचक्षते । तेजोध्यानाल्लक्षगुणं सूक्ष्मध्यानं परात्परम् ॥२२

sthūladhyānācchataguṇam tejodhyānaṃ pracakṣate |

tejodhyānāllakṣaguṇaṃ sūkṣmadhyānaṃ parātparam ॥ 22

6.22 the scriptures say that a hundred times superior to idol worship is the meditation on inner light, or chakra meditation.

And one lakh times more effective than luminous meditation is the subtle vibrations meditation, that is only switched ON by the Guru.

Note that both luminous and subtle vibration meditations are given by Guru alone, and these may be interchanged by Him to suit the disciples in accordance with the general state of evolution in the current time period.

इति ते कथितं चण्ड ध्यानयोगं सुदुर्लभम् । आत्मा साक्षाद्भवेद्यस्मात्तस्माद्ध्यानं विशिष्यते

॥२३॥ iti te kathitaṃ caṇḍa dhyānayogaṃ sudurlabham |

ātmā sākṣādbhavedyasmāttasmāddhyānaṃ viśiṣyate ॥ 23

6.22 O effulgent seeker! This have Thee learnt the ultimate techniques of Meditation, which only rare Masters teach, and rarer still grasp.

Meditation is the only way to have a glimpse of the ultimate reality, and even once having had this touch, you shall always be protected, cared for, and talented.

॥ इति श्रीघेरण्डसंहितायां घेरण्डचण्डसंवादे घटस्थयोगे सप्तसाधने ध्यानयोगो नाम

षष्ठोपदेशः ॥ iti śrīgheraṇḍasaṃhitāyāṃ gheraṇḍacaṇḍasaṃvāde

ghaṭasthayoge saptasādhane dhyānayogo nāma ṣaṣṭhopadeśaḥ ॥

Thus ends the 6th Chapter.

7 Dissolving - Samadhi समाधियोगो नाम सप्तमोपदेशः

घेरण्ड उवाच । gheraṇḍa uvāca । समाधिश्च परो योगो बहुभाग्येन लभ्यते । गुरोः कृपाप्रसादेन प्राप्यते गुरुभक्तितः ॥ १ ॥ samādhiśca paro yogo bahubhāgyena labhyate । guroḥ kṛpāprasādena prāpyate gurubhaktitaḥ ॥ 1

7.1 the sage goes on to eulogize the Guru. A Guru comes in one's life only by great good fortune. The company of a Guru is the best thing to happen in a human life. No amount of wealth, power or fame can deliver what a Guru delivers.

An intense yearning to know the truth, to seek the transcendental is the prerequisite.

The 3 challenges

विद्याप्रतीतिः स्वगुरुप्रतीतिरात्मप्रतीतिर्मनसः प्रबोधः ।
दिने दिने यस्य भवेत्स योगी सुशोभनाभ्यासमुपैति सद्यः ॥ २

vidyāpratītiḥ svagurupratītirātmapratītirmanasaḥ prabodhaḥ ।

dine dine yasya bhavetsa yogī suśobhanābhyāsamupaiti sadyaḥ ॥ 2

7.2 there are the three challenges one faces on this path. 1) is the knowledge adequate? 2) am I qualified to receive the teaching? 3) is the Master genuine and can he help me?

An enthusiastic faith in the techniques, a steady faith in oneself, and a deep faith in the Guru help one overcome these subtle yet difficult concerns.

The process is long drawn, the wisdom gets filtered in slowly yet surely day by day.

घटाद्भिन्नं मनः कृत्वा ऐक्यं कुर्यात्परात्मनि ।समाधिं तं विजानीयान्मुक्तसंज्ञो दशादिभिः ॥३

ghaṭādbhinnam manaḥ kṛtvā aikyam kuryātparātmani ।

samādhim tam vijānīyānmuktasaṃjño daśādibhiḥ ॥ 3

7.3 Again and again tell yourself "asangho hum", you are not the body, you are not the mind, nor the impressions.

There is the pure, untouched divine spark inside you, know that you are part of God. You have it within you to transcend all grief, overcome any failure, and become happy and blissful.

अहं ब्रह्म न चान्योऽस्मि ब्रह्मैवाहं न शोकभाक् । सच्चिदानन्दरूपोऽहं नित्यमुक्तः स्वभाववान् ॥ ४ ॥ aham brahma na cānyo'smi brahmaivāham na

śokabhāk | saccidānandarūpo'ham nityamuktaḥ svabhāvavān || 4
7.4 I am Brahman, I am not other. Hear the
Brahmagyanvali mala of Adi Sankara.
I am sachidananda, I am free from guilt and grief, I am one with the divine.

शाम्भव्या चैव भ्रामर्या खेचर्या योनिमुद्रया । ध्यानं नादं रसानन्दं लयसिद्धिश्चतुर्विधा ॥ ५

sāmbhavyā caiva bhrāmaryā khecaryā yonimudrayā |

dhyānam nādam rasānandam layasiddhiścaturvidhā || 5
7.5 the blissful dissolution is of four types - attained by dhyana - visualisation, nada- sacred sounds, rasa - taste buds, and laya - any other sense being merged in the infinite.

The prior practice of Yogic techniques taught earlier, including Shambhavi, Khechari, Brahmari and Yoni mudras, are quite helpful in achieving the same.

पञ्चधा भक्तियोगेन मनोमूर्च्छा च षड्विधा । षड्विधोऽयं राजयोगः प्रत्येकमवधारयेत् ॥ ६

pañcadhā bhaktiyogena manomūrcchā ca ṣaḍvidhā |

ṣaḍvidho'yam rājayogaḥ pratyekamavadhārayet || 6
7.6 The fifth type of blissful dissolution is the one got from living a life of devotion.
The sixth type of Samadhi is the one attained by hardships and direct experience of Sages who negate all shallowness, but this

path is extremely painful and not recommended for all.

अथ ध्यानयोगसमाधिः । atha dhyānayogasamādhiḥ ।

शाम्भवीं मुद्रिकां कृत्वा आत्मप्रत्यक्षमानयेत् ।बिन्दु ब्रह्ममयं दृष्ट्वा मनस्तत्र नियोजयेत् ॥७

śāmbhavīṃ mudrikāṃ kṛtvā ātmapratyakṣamānayet ।

bindu brahmamayaṃ dṛṣṭvā manastatra niyojayet ॥ 7

7.7 now the master guides us through various practical examples of achieving blissful dissolution.

A technique is mentioned of visualisation by employing Shambhavi Mudra and fixing one's focus on a tiny point inside the brain between the eyebrows. It can lead to Dhyana Samadhi.

खमध्ये कुरु चात्मानमात्ममध्ये च खं कुरु । आत्मानं खमयं दृष्ट्वा न किञ्चिदपि बाधते ।

सदानन्दमयो भूत्वा समाधिस्थो भवेन्नरः ॥ ८

ātmānaṃ khamayaṃ dṛṣṭvā na kiñcidapi bādhate ।

sadānandamayo bhūtvā samādhistho bhavennaraḥ ॥ 8

7.8 another technique - experience the space all around oneself in the room one is sitting in, and identify the hollow and empty space within one's body.
Soon one's mind dissolves and Samadhi is experienced.

अथ नादयोगसमाधिः । atha nādayogasamādhiḥ ।

अनिलं मन्दवेगेन भ्रामरीकुम्भकं चरेत् । मन्दं मन्दं रेचयेद्वायुं भृङ्गनादं ततो भवेत् ॥ ९

anilaṃ mandavegena bhrāmarīkumbhakaṃ caret ।

mandaṃ mandaṃ recayedvāyuṃ bhṛṅganādaṃ tato bhavet ॥ 9

7.9 another technique - we do Brahmari gradually humming like a bee for a few times,

अन्तःस्थं भ्रमरीनादं श्रुत्वा तत्र मनो नयेत् । समाधिर्जायते तत्र आनन्दः सोऽहमित्यतः ॥१०

antaḥstham bhramarīnādaṃ śrutvā tatra mano nayet |

samādhirjāyate tatra ānandaḥ so'hamityataḥ || 10

7.10 and our mind hears the sound vibration in the ears and brain, and the whole body slowly gets detached from the surroundings. We experience a blissful state. The Soham state means the same, That bliss is Me.

अथ रसनानन्दयोगसमाधिः । खेचरीमुद्रासाधनाद्रसनोर्ध्वगता यदा । तदा समाधिसिद्धिः स्याद्धित्वा साधारणक्रियाम् ॥ ११ ॥ atha rasanānandayogasamādhiḥ |

khecarīmudrāsādhanādrasanordhvagatā yadā | tadā samādhisiddhiḥ

syāddhitvā sādhāraṇakriyām || 11

7.11 another technique - use khechari mudra, rub or touch lightly the top of the palate with the tongue, soon the senses become balanced, the emotions lose their grip, and samadhi is experienced.

अथ लयसिद्धियोगसमाधिः । atha layasiddhiyogasamādhiḥ |

योनिमुद्रां समासाद्य स्वयं शक्तिमयो भवेत् । सुशृङ्गाररसेनैव विहरेत्परमात्मनि ॥ १२

yonimudrāṃ samāsādya svayaṃ śaktimayo bhavet |

suśaṛṅgārarasenaiva viharetparamātmani || 12

7.12 again by doing the Yoni Mudra, one can experience a union of oneself with one's beloved, for a while one becomes dissolved in that.

आनन्दमयः सम्भूत्वा ऐक्यं ब्रह्मणि सम्भवेत् ।अहं ब्रह्मेति चाऽद्वैतं समाधिस्तेन जायते ॥

१३ ॥ ānandamayaḥ sambhūtvā aikyaṃ brahmaṇi sambhavet | ahaṃ

brahmeti cā'dvaitaṃ samādhistena jāyate || 13

7.13 a great joy is got in such union, as the bliss of uniting with the divine.
A sense of victorious peace pervades, aham Brahma - I am brahman.
Such states of dissolution are the states of Advaita or non-duality. They erase all sorrow, fill renewed hope, stamina is restored, and

life moves up the evolutionary ladder.

अथ भक्तियोगसमाधिः । atha bhaktiyogasamādhiḥ ।

स्वकीयहृदये ध्यायेदिष्टदेवस्वरूपकम् । चिन्तयेद्भक्तियोगेन परमाह्लादपूर्वकम् ॥ १४

svakīyahṛdaye dhyāyediṣṭadevasvarūpakam ।

cintayedbhaktiyogena paramāhlādapūrvakam ॥ 14

7.14 for a bhakta, life is a continuous service of his divine. Singing, glorifying, listening to stories of his lord, he easily passes into states of dissolution.

आनन्दाश्रुपुलकेन दशाभावः प्रजायते । समाधिः सम्भवेत्तेन सम्भवेच्च मनोन्मनी ॥ १५

ānandāśrupulakena daśābhāvaḥ prajāyate ।

samādhiḥ sambhavettena sambhavecca manonmanī ॥ 15

7.15 his eyes shed tears of gratefulness, his breath chants the divine name at work and play.

अथ राजयोगसमाधिः । atha rājayogasamādhiḥ ।

मनोमूर्च्छां समासाद्य मन आत्मनि योजयेत् । परात्मनः समायोगात्समाधि समवाप्नुयात्

॥ १६ ॥ manomūrcchāṃ samāsādya mana ātmani yojayet ।

parātmanaḥ samāyogātsamādhiṃ samavāpnuyāt ॥ 16

7.16 for the intellectual giant the process is of continuous negation, not this not this, and this makes him dazed and he goes into a trance after much effort.

अथ समाधियोगमाहात्म्यम् । atha samādhiyogamāhātmyam ।

इति ते कथितं चण्ड समाधिर्मुक्तिलक्षणम्। राजयोगः समाधिः स्यादेकात्मन्येव साधनम् ।

उन्मनी सहजावस्था सर्वे चैकात्मवाचकाः ॥ १७

iti te kathitaṃ caṇḍa samādhirmuktilakṣaṇam ।

rājayogaḥ samādhiḥ syādekātmanyeva sādhanam ।

unmanī sahajāvasthā sarve caikātmavācakāḥ ॥ 17

7.17 o calm and earnest seeker! thus have I taught thee the ultimate means of attaining freedom.

The Raja yoga or the king's path of separating the chaff from the kernel, and the Sahaj or easy path that most can tread, all lead to the divine. Practice what you please, and attain ultimate and permanent bliss.

जले विष्णुः स्थले विष्णुर्विष्णुः पर्वतमस्तके । ज्वालामालाकुले विष्णुः सर्वं विष्णुमयं जगत् ॥ १८ ॥ jale viṣṇuḥ sthale viṣṇurviṣṇuḥ parvatamastake |

jvālāmālākule viṣṇuḥ sarvaṃ viṣṇumayaṃ jagat ॥ 18
7.18 know that all of creation is pervaded by the Lord. He is there in the oceans, he fills the valleys, he covers the mountain tops.

Volcanoes and volcanic ash contain him, he is present in all of us as well.

भूचराः खेचराश्चामी यावन्तो जीवजन्तवः । वृक्षगुल्मलतावल्लीतृणाद्या वारिपर्वताः । सर्वं ब्रह्म विजानीयात्सर्वं पश्यति चात्मनि ॥ १९ ॥ bhūcarāḥ khecarāścāmī

yāvanto jīvajantavaḥ | vṛkṣagulmalatāvallītṛṇādyā vāriparvatāḥ |

sarvaṃ brahma vijānīyātsarvaṃ paśyati cātmani ॥ 19
7.19 all animals who roam the dry plains, all birds who love to fly, all living beings are his domain.

Trees, plants, creepers, vines and grass, whether on land or in the oceans, know them all to be divine.

See the divine in all beings and in all things.

आत्मा घटस्थचैतन्यमद्वैतं शाश्वतं परम् । घटाद्विभिन्नतो ज्ञात्वा वीतरागं विवासनम् ॥२०
ātmā ghaṭasthacaitanyamadvaitaṃ śāśvataṃ param |

ghaṭādvibhinnato jñātvā vītarāgaṃ vivāsanam ॥ 20
7.20 understand that there is a soul inside this mechanical clay-pot like anatomical body.

That soul is the spark of the divine, which is non-dual, eternal, and everyone's ultimate aim.

Make the divine your prime target, different yet not different from this perishable body, separate yet not separate with these subtle thoughts and emotions.

एवं मिथः समाधिः स्यात्सर्वसङ्कल्पवर्जितः । स्वदेहे पुत्रदारादिबान्धवेषु धनादिषु ।
सर्वेषु निर्ममो भूत्वा समाधि समवाप्नुयात् ॥ २१

svadehe putradārādibāndhaveṣu dhanādiṣu |

sarveṣu nirmamo bhūtvā samādhiṃ samavāpnuyāt || 21
7.21 the same is your experience in samadhi. When you dissociate from your limitations.

Samadhi is the state of oneness, you are no longer limited or hijacked or thwarted by your body, your children, your beloved, your friends, your colleagues, or your assets.

This state of not feeling the pressure, nor the stress and strain is called Samadhi.

तत्त्वं लयामृतं गोप्यं शिवोक्तं विविधानि च । तेषां सङ्क्षेपमादाय कथितं मुक्तिलक्षणम् ॥२२

tattvaṃ layāmṛtaṃ gopyaṃ śivoktaṃ vividhāni ca |

teṣāṃ saṅkṣepamādāya kathitaṃ muktilakṣaṇam || 22
7.22 the wise and benevolent sages have taught various techniques to their disciples.

I have learnt from them and taught you a handful. However these are sufficient for your emancipation. You shall surely attain your aims and the ultimate freedom by a diligent practice of these.

इति ते कथितं चण्ड समाधिर्दुर्लभः परः । यं ज्ञात्वा न पुनर्जन्म जायते भूमिमण्डले ॥ २३

iti te kathitaṃ caṇḍa samādhirdurlabhaḥ paraḥ |

yaṃ jñātvā na punarjanma jāyate bhūmimaṇḍale || 23

7.23 o reverential and sincere seeker, thus have you experienced Meditation, that which is the hardest to experience.

By this experience of deep meditation or samadhi, there is no getting caught in traps of guilt and suffering.

Life becomes a thrill, the journey becomes infused with divine charms and all is taken care of admirably.

|| इति श्रीघेरण्डसंहितायां घेरण्डयोगेश्वरनृपचण्डकापालिसंवादे घटस्थयोगसाधने योगस्य सप्तसारे समाधियोगो नाम सप्तमोपदेशः समाप्तः || iti śrīgheraṇḍasaṃhitāyāṃ gheraṇḍayogeśvaranṛpacaṇḍakāpāli-saṃvāde ghaṭasthayogasādhane yogasya saptasāre samādhiyogo nāma saptamopadeśaḥ samāptaḥ ||

End of the famous Dialogue that has laid the foundation for all forms of Yoga as it is being practiced today in various schools. Om Svasti.

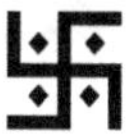

Before Beginning

Some preparations done beforehand deepen the satisfaction and make it rewarding.

Pleasantly Lit, Well Ventilated Room

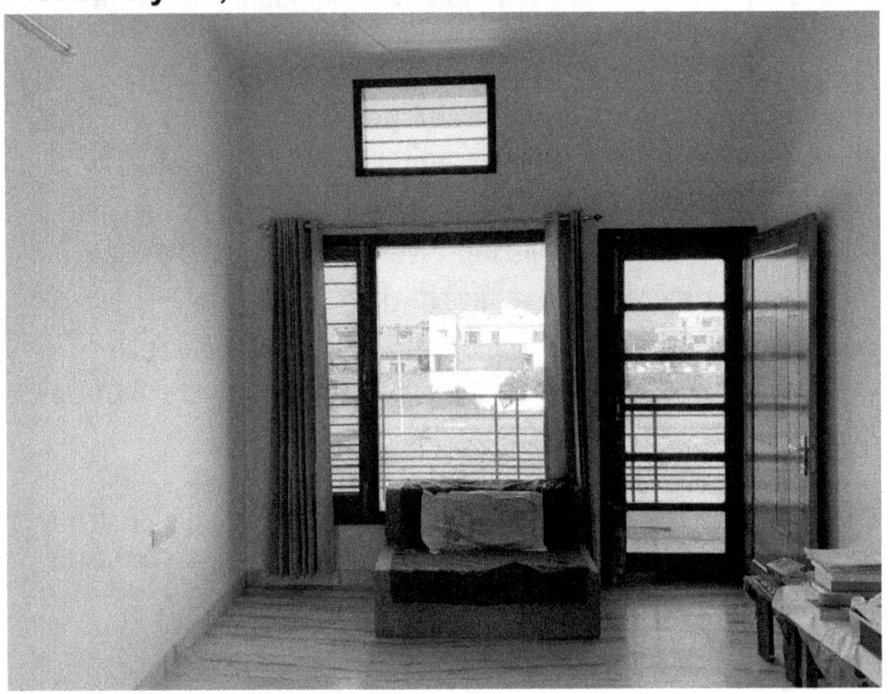

Yoga Mat and Water Bottle

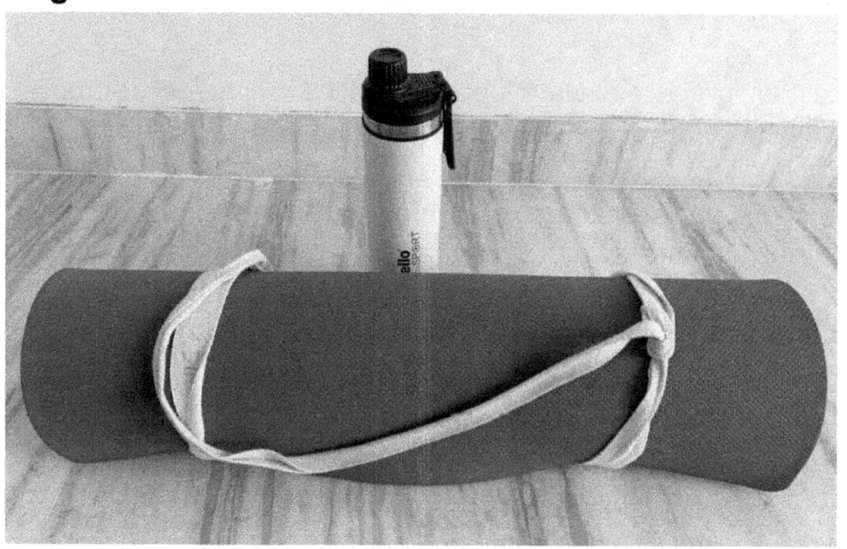

Begin with a Gratefulness

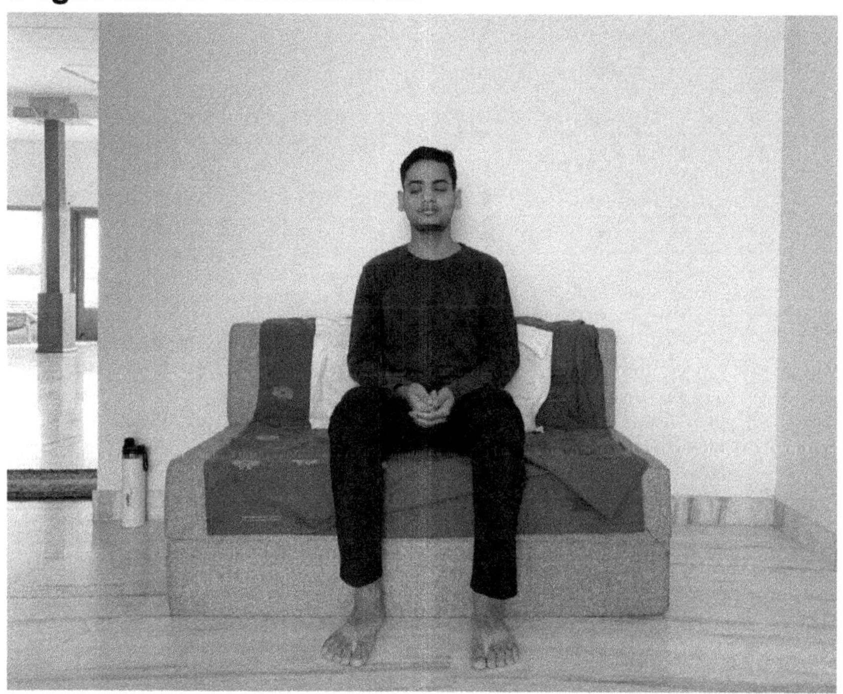

Warm Ups

It is a good practice to warm up a bit by a walk, light jog, or simply moving the joints of the neck, shoulder, and ankle a few times.

A very good pelvic opener, thighs, hips, and knees relaxer is the Butterfly Dynamic Pose.

For massaging the Spine, try the Cat Stretch Dynamic Pose.

A quick and easy whole body loosener is the Bridge Pose.

Making Rain with the Arms n Palms
Blinking the Eyes
Massaging the Ears
Take good care of yourself
REGULARLY

BRIDGE

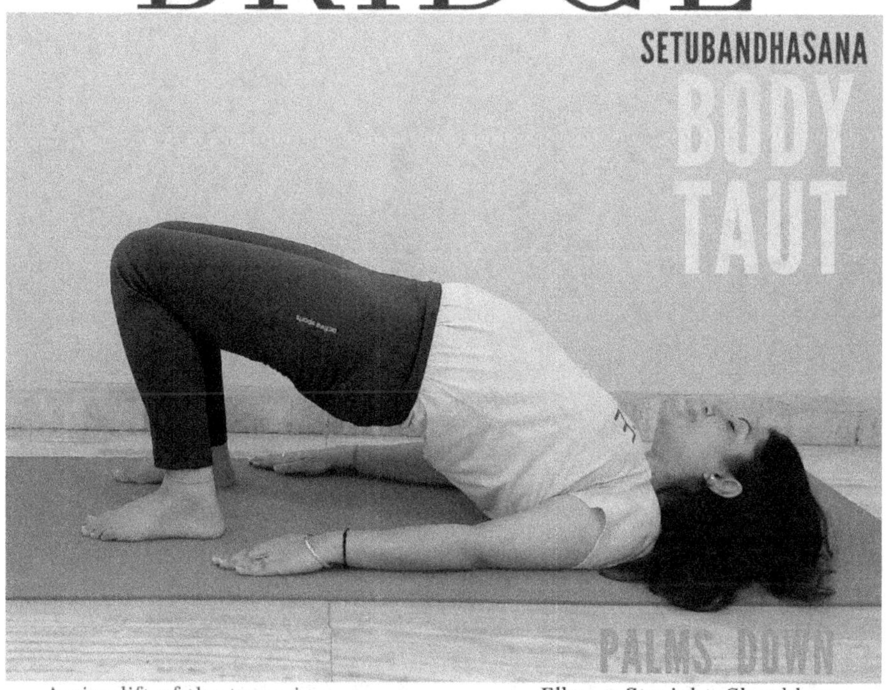

A nice lift of the torso in a gentle sloping arch. Feet firmly planted.

Elbows Straight. Shoulders anchored

NECK FIRM

Maintain focus on lumbar low back, make each breath smooth s l o w quiver-free

POSE FOR 6 BREATHS

BUTTERFLY

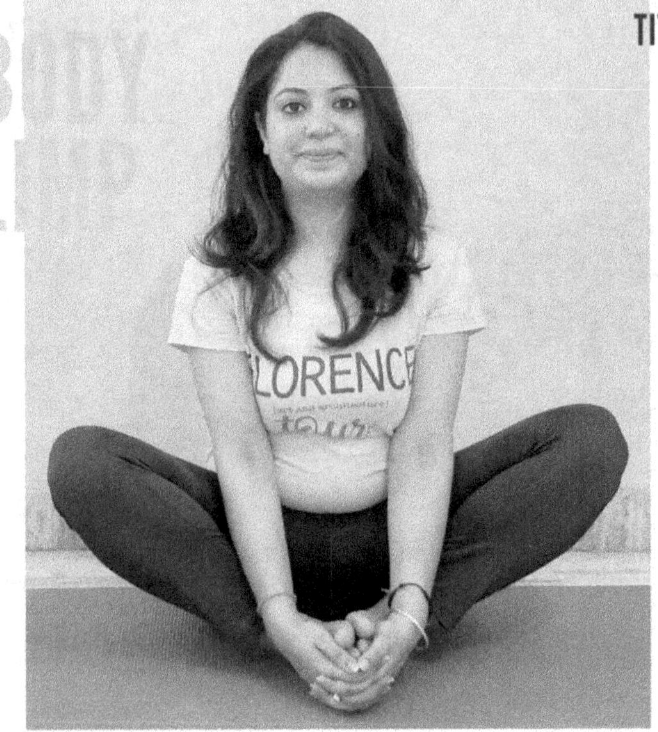

FLAP THE LEGS MIMIC A BUTTERFLY

FLY CHEERFULLY FOR 2 MINUTES

PRONE
VISHNU

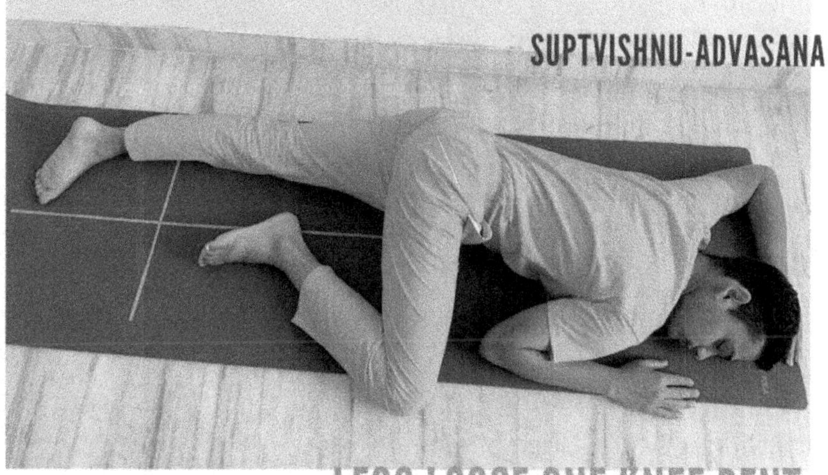

LEGS LOOSE ONE KNEE BENT

Neck loose. Face Relaxed.
Delicate sleep

BODY LIMP

PALMS OPEN TO FLOOR

Let go the focus, make
each breath smooth s l o w
quiver-free

POSE AS LONG AS COMFORTABLE

Yoga Nidra

We look for so much attention outside. We go crazy trying to please someone. In our Yogic tradition there is a brilliant method of taking a conscious shower that harmonizes each body part and actually raises our charm to a degree that cosmetics and body sprays can never do.

Remember –
- the key to efficient performance at the workplace
- the magic in engaging relationships

is deep and sufficient relaxation.

Yog Nidra Sadhguru Guided Meditation for Sleep
https://www.youtube.com/watch?v=veeAGGq577s

Yoga Nidra - Guided Meditation for Sleep & Relaxation – Sri Sri
https://www.youtube.com/watch?v=zLJu3wQA1Ko

Yoga Nidra - Swami Niranjanananda Saraswati
https://www.youtube.com/watch?v=04qZCaKFSWc

Meditation

It goes without saying that Meditation twice a day for a few minutes shall integrate and bind all our activities, enhance our immunity greatly, and lead to long term material success that is stable.

Meditation is simply honoring the unknown. Getting in touch with the cosmos, the infinite vastness that fulfills all and showers pleasurable bliss.

Memory and Meditation –
A Neuroscientist in Conversation with Sri Sri
https://www.youtube.com/watch?v=h7lPFXJCvKI

Meditate with Gurudev
https://www.srisriravishankar.org/live/
https://www.youtube.com/playlist?list=PLH-0HZ0SQ_PEYRcjsRvxivVhGPk2iT6iZ

10-minute Guided Meditation for Beginners
https://www.youtube.com/watch?v=TWbiDzi-rQc

Glow of the Candle
https://www.youtube.com/watch?v=-vrcUArnd-w

Meditate with your Breath
https://www.youtube.com/watch?v=SShjEQfK-w0

Healing Flute Music
https://www.youtube.com/watch?v=unuiaZleQ5c

Technology of Spirituality – A talk by Khurshed Batliwala
https://www.youtube.com/watch?v=l9aR_xfm-gE

After Ending

May lie down in Shavasana

Eyes closed.
Loosen and adjust all joints and muscles. Then become still. Make the breath soft.

Rest as long as needed. Then roll to the right side and sit up.

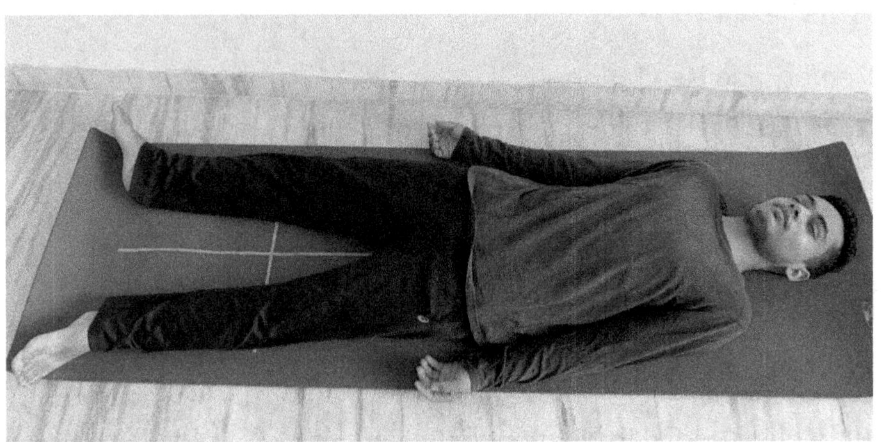

Grace is in Gratefulness

Smile freely. Offer your practice to the Great Lord. To your near and dear ones. And become Free.

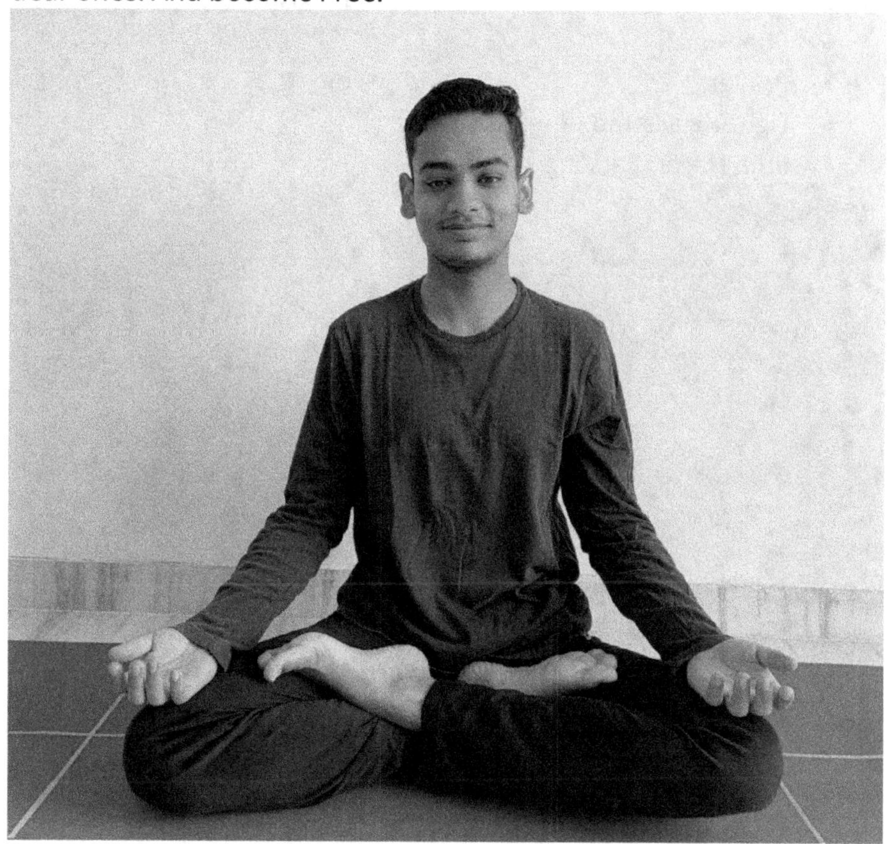

Regular Habits

Apart from asana practice, the following habits support our Yoga aura and nurture us from a deeper plane of existence.

- Chanting
- Prayer
- Lighting a Lamp
- Puja Havan Satsang Aarti

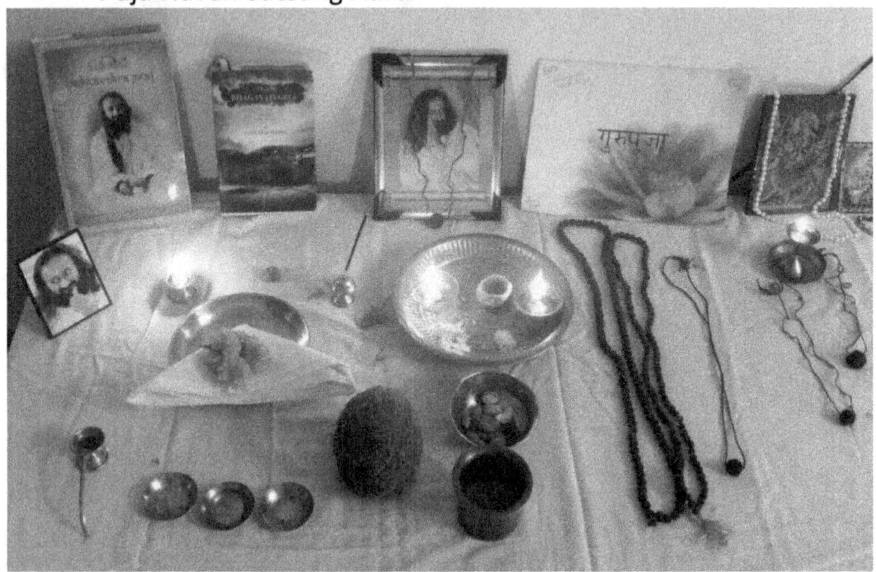

Guruji answers - Why is Puja Necessary?
https://www.youtube.com/watch?v=PuFqCrl8SX0

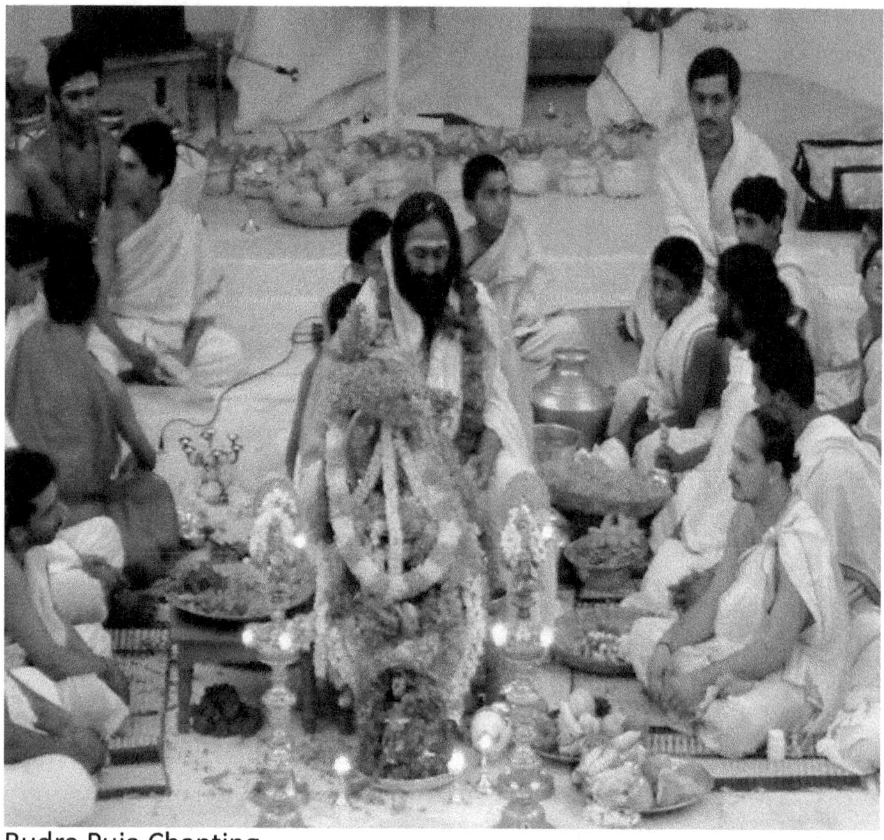

Rudra Puja Chanting
https://www.youtube.com/watch?v=QjsO4UVwsow

Guru Puja by Bhanu Didi
https://www.youtube.com/watch?v=htXI6Fommfw

Daily Watch

Food is a potential parameter that can make or break any target. For some reason, the scientific reasons behind eating a proper vegetarian diet has been long forgotten or overlooked. However, it is slowly surfacing and being talked about in the medical circles and journals. Famous personalities are boldly implementing it, and their success is enough testimony for the same.

Ayurveda & Diet

Ayurveda is a safe mechanism to mix and match our diet as per our native constitution. It will prevent many ills and mood swings. It makes sense to get a pulse diagnosis nadi pariksha done. And it goes without saying that locally grown fresh fruits and vegetables, and A2 cow milk products should be a diet priority. Replacing white sugar with honey, jaggery, etc., sea salt with rock salt, and refined oils with cold pressed mustard or groundnut oil, such culinary methods make a remarkable turnaround in overall health levels.
https://www.artofliving.org/ayurveda

Vitamins

Due to the increased usage of mechanized farming, packaged foods, and high dosage of chemicals, colors, preservatives, or flavors in our eatables, the real essence of food is pushed far into the background. It just remains a belly fill without nourishment. So, we must supplement our diet with Shakti Drops and other Ayurvedic concoctions.

Gurudev on Turmeric and Ginger and Giloye (Amruth balli)
https://www.youtube.com/watch?v=sYoCdmjkGlg

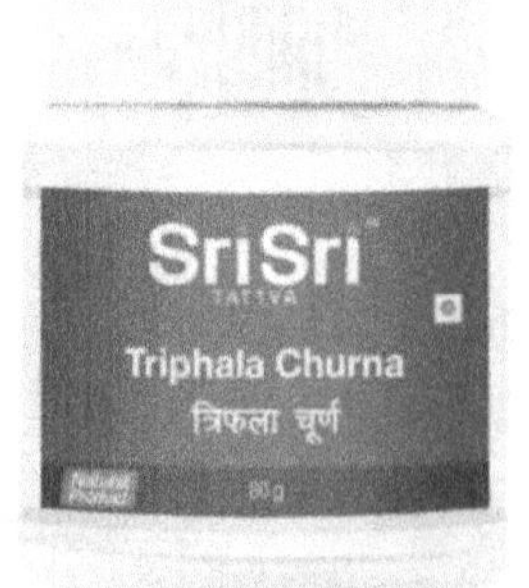

Eat a teaspoon of Triphala Churna with warm water at bedtime for a fortnight.

Wash your eyes daily with Triphala water for ten days.

Eye Care & Tooth Care

Eyes are most beautiful and need to be kept functional till a ripe old age. We can wash them with triphala water that has been strained using a fine cloth. Simply add a teaspoon of triphala powder to a cup of plain water and leave overnight in a copper vessel.

Also, keep a tissue paper dipped in cool Rose water over the eyes and relax for a few minutes with eyes closed.

Sri Sri Shakti Drops
It is advisable to add 4 drops to a cup of water and drink regularly.
https://www.amazon.in/Sri-Ayurveda-Shakti-Drops-10/dp/B017IJGG44

Patanjali Dant Kanti Manjan
https://www.patanjaliayurved.net/product/natural-personal-care/dental-care/advanced-dant-kanti-manjan/870

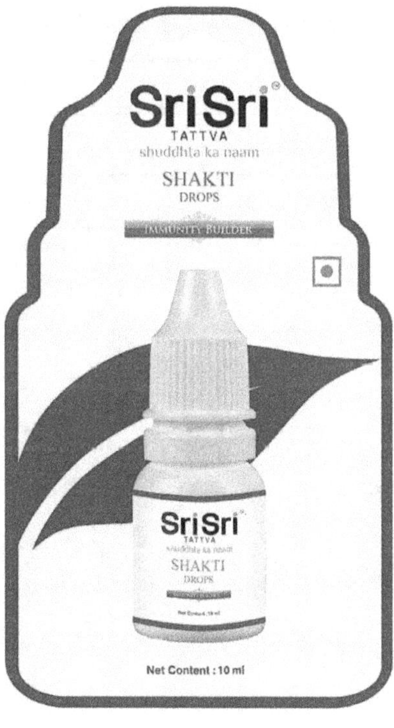

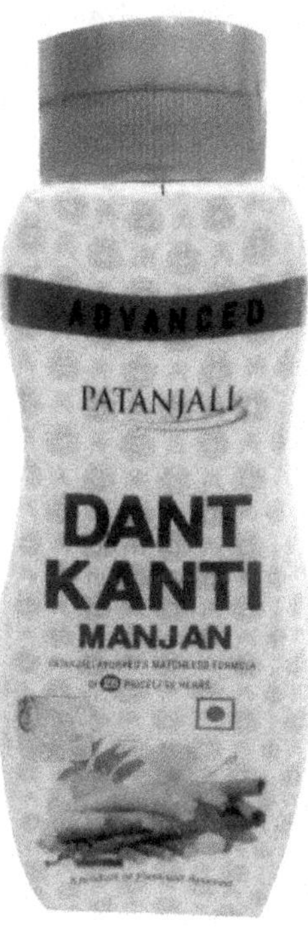

Keeping healthy teeth and gums is no longer possible by regular brushing alone due to a drastic intake of packaged and fast foods. Daily dant manjan is a must.

Latin Transliteration Chart

International Alphabet of Sanskrit Transliteration (I.A.S.T.)

a	ā	i	ī	u	ū	r̥	r̥̄	l̥	
अ	आ	इ	ई	उ	ऊ	ऋ	ॠ	ऌ	
						ृ	ॄ	ॢ	
e	ai	o	au	ṃ	m̐	ḥ	Ardha Visarga	oṃ	
ए	ऐ	ओ	औ	◌ं	◌ँ	◌:	ꣳ	ॐ	

Consonants are shown with a vowel 'a= अ' for uttering

ka	क	ca	च	ṭa	ट	ta	त	pa	प
kha	ख	cha	छ	ṭha	ठ	tha	थ	pha	फ
ga	ग	ja	ज	ḍa	ड	da	द	ba	ब
gha	घ	jha	झ	ḍha	ढ	dha	ध	bha	भ
ṅa	ङ	ña	ञ	ṇa	ण	na	न	ma	म
ya	ra	la	va		ḷa	'			
य	र	ल	व		ळ	S			

				Consonant only		
śa	ṣa	sa	ha		ka	क्अ = क
श	ष	स	ह		k	क्

Alphabetical Index of Techniques

Shatkarma – Bathing / Body Parts and Organs Cleansing

Sanskrit Name	English	Verse	SN
Agnisara Dhauti	Stomach	1.20	1
Danta Dhauti	Teeth	1.26 - 27	3
Danta Moola Dhauti	Gums/Root of Teeth	1.28	4
Hrida Basti	Food Pipe/Throat	1.36 - 37	8
Jihva Dhauti	Tongue	1.29	5
Kapalarandhra	Sinuses	1.34	7
Kapalbhati	Forehead/Sinuses	1.55 -59	12
Karna Dhauti	Ears	1.33	6
Lauliki	Diaphragm	1.52	10
Neti	Nostrils	1.50 - 51	9
Shankh Prakshalana	Stomach/Colon	1.23 - 24	2
Trataka	Eyes	1.53 – 54	11

Asana – Posture / Body Alignment

Sanskrit Name	English	Verse	SN
Bhadrasana	Strength	2.9-10	3
Bhujangasana	Cobra	2.42-43	31
Dhanurasana	Bow	2.18	10
Garudasana	Eagle	2.37	26
Gomukhasana	Cow's Face	2.16	8
Gorakshasana	Cowherd	2.25-26	16
Guptasana	Hidden	2.2	12
Kukkatsana	Rooster	2.31	20
Kurmasana	Tortoise	2.32	21
Makarasana	Crocodile	2.4	29
Mandukasana	Frog	2.34	23
Matsyasana	Fish	2.21	13
Matsyendrasana	Lord of Fish	2.22-23	14
Mayurasana	Peacock	2.29-30	19

Muktasana / Sukhasana	Freedom	2.11	4
Padmasana	Lotus	2.8	2
Paschimottanasana	Back Stretch	2.24	15
Sankatasana	Danger	2.28	18
Shalabhasana	Locust	2.39	28
Shavasana	Corpse	2.19	11
Siddhasana	Perfect Pose	2.7	1
Simhasana	Lion	2.14-15	7
Swastikasana	Auspicious	2.13	6
Ushtrasana	Camel	2.41	30
Utkatasana	Chair	2.27	17
Uttana Kurmasana	Raised Tortoise	2.33	22
Uttana Mandukasana	Raised Frog	2.35	24
Vajrasana	Thunderbolt	2.12	5
Virasana	Brave	2.17	9
Vrikshasana	Tree	2.36	25
Vrishabasana / Vrishasana	Bull	2.38	27
Yogasana	Yogic	2.44-45	32

Pranayama – Breath Regulation / Breathing Consciously

Sanskrit Name	English	Verse	
Nadi Shodhana	Alternate Nostril Breathing	5.39 - 45	
Bija यं	With Seed sound "yam"	5.40	
Bija रं	Seed sound "ram"	5.41 – 42	
Bija ठं	Seed sound "tham"	5.43 - 44	
Bija वं	Seed sound "vam"	5.43 - 44	
Bija लं	Seed sound "lam"	5.43 - 44	
Matra	Breath Counting	5.55	
Suryabheda	Heating Breath	5.66	
Ujjayi	Victory over Senses	5.69 - 70	
Shitali	Cooling Breath	5.73 - 74	

Bhastrika	Bellows Breath	5.75 - 77	
Brahmari	Humming OM	5.78 - 80	
Murccha	Dazed orFainting	5.83	
Soham / Kevali	Rhythmic Breathing	5.84 - 96	

Mudra – Gesture / Hand Sign

Sanskrit Name	English	Verse	SN
Ashwini Mudra	Horse	3.82 - 83	16
Bhujangini Mudra	Serpent	3.92 - 93	20
Kaki Mudra	Crow	3.86 - 87	18
Khechari Mudra	Five Senses	3.25 - 32	8
Maha Mudra	Great	3.6 - 8	1
Manduki Mudra	Frog	3.62 - 63	14
Matangini Mudra	Elephant	3.88 - 91	19
Nabho Mudra	Navel	3.9	2
Pashini Mudra	Posterior	3.84 - 85	17
Shaktichalani	Kundalini	3.49 - 60	12
Shambhavi Mudra	Third Eye	3.64 - 67	15
Tadagi Mudra	Abdomen	3.61	13
Vajroli Mudra	Thunderbolt	3.45 - 48	11
Viparitkarni Mudra	Reversal	3.33 - 36	9
Yoni Mudra	Union	3.37 - 44	10

Bandha – Lock / Sealing the exit of wind

Sanskrit Name	English	Verse	SN
Jalandhar Bandha	Neck Seal	3.12 - 13	2
Maha Bandha	Great Seal	3.18 - 20	4
Maha Vedha Mudra	Intense Sealing Gesture	3.21 - 24	5
Moola Bandha	Anus Seal	3.14 - 17	3
Uddiyana Bandha	Diaphragm Seal	3.10 - 11	1

Pratyahara – Inward U turn

Sanskrit Name	English	Verse	SN
Manas Chanchalam	Thoughts, Memory triggers	4.2	1
Manas Drishti	Sight awareness	4.3	2
Manas Ghrana	Odors awareness	4.6	5
Manas Rasam	Tongue and Taste awareness	4.7	6
Manas Shravanam	Hearing and Speech awareness	4.4	3
Manas Sparsha	Touch, Atmosphere awareness	4.5	4

Dharana – Fixed Focus

Sanskrit Name	English	Verse	SN
Adho Dharana, Bija लं	Earth Imagination	3.70-71	1
Ambhasi Dharana, Bija वं	Water Imagination	3.72-74	2
Vaishvanari Dharana, Bija रं	Fire Imagination	3.75-76	3
Vayavi Dharana, Bija यं	Air Imagination	3.77-79	4
Vyoma Dharana, Bija हं	Space Imagination	3.80-81	5

Dhyana – Meditation (some examples listed)

Sanskrit Name	English	Verse	SN
Jyotis Dhyana	Luminous Meditation	6.12	2
Sthula Dhyana	Deity/Chanting Meditation	6.2	1
Sukshama Dhyana	Vibration/Feeling Meditation	6.13	3

Samadhi – Dissolution (example combinations told)

Sanskrit Name	English	Verse	SN
Bhakti Yoga Samadhi	Dissolving by Glorifying	7.14 - 15	5
Dhyana Samadhi	Dissolving by Third Eye Focus	7.7 - 8	1
Laya Samadhi	Dissolving by Union	7.12 - 13	4
Nada Samadhi	Dissolving by Senses Restraint	7.9	2
Raja Yoga Samadhi	Dissolving by Negation	7.16	6
Rasa Ananda Samadhi	Dissolving by Chanting	7.10 - 11	3

References

https://www.ashtangayoga.info/philosophy/sanskrit-and-devanagari/transliteration-tool/

http://www.sarahburgessyoga.com/about-yoga/
https://www.classicyoga.co.in/
https://srisrischoolofyoga.org/in/
Baba Ramdev https://www.youtube.com/watch?v=76JRRnUfTl0

Srisa Chandra Vasu – The Gheranda Samhita – 1st – 1914 – Reprint 1979 Sri Satguru Publications, Delhi.

Swami Satyananda Saraswati – A Systematic Course in the Ancient Tantric Techniques of Yoga and Kriya – 1st – 1981 – Reprint 2013 - Yoga Publications Trust, Munger.

Swami Mahesananda – Jogapradipyaka – 1st – 2006 – Kaivalyadhama S.M.Y.M. Samiti, Lonavla.

Swami Mahesananda – Vasistha Samhita – 3rd – 2018 – Kaivalyadhama S.M.Y.M. Samiti, Lonavla.

Swami Kuvalayananda – Goraksa Satakam – Reprint 2019 – Kaivalyadhama, Pune.

Yoga Yajnavalkya Samhita – Revised 2015 – Krishnamacharya Yoga Mandiram, Chennai.

B K S Iyengar– Light on Yoga – 1st – 1966 – Reprint 2020 - HarperCollins Publishers, India.

Yoga in Daily Life – 7th – 1998 – Institute of Naturopathy & Yogic Sciences, Bangalore.

M L Gharote – Hatharatnavali of Srinivasa Yogi– 1st – 2002 – Reprint 2019 – The Lonavla Yoga Institute, Lonavla.

Swami Satyananda Saraswati – Asana Pranayama Mudra Bandha –
1st – 1966 – Revised 1999 – Bihar School of Yoga, Munger.

Swami Muktibodhananda – Hatha Yoga Pradipika – 3rd – 1998 –
Yoga Publications Trust, Munger.

Swami Niranjanananda Saraswati – Gheranda Samhita – 1st – 2012 –
Yoga Publications Trust, Munger.

Ashwini Kumar Aggarwal, Devotees of Sri Sri Ravi Shankar Ashram,
Punjab, Publications.
– Bhagavad Gita Applied Wisdom – 1st – 2018.
– Patanjali Yoga Sutras: Essence and Sanskrit Grammar – 1st – 2018.
– Prashna Upanishad: Essence and Sanskrit Grammar – 1st – 2020.
– Sanskrit Past Participles Nishtha – 1st – 2020.
– YOGA Science and Practice – 1st – 2020.

Epilogue

Sudarshan Kriya as taught by Gurudev Sri Sri Ravi Shankar is the
ultimate technique for Yoga in daily life. It beautifully covers all
aspects to keep fit as outlined in Gheranda Samhita and is followed
by millions around the globe in 156 countries.

And who qualifies for Sudarshan Kriya Yoga, aptly abbreviated as
SKY? Anyone above the age of 18 years, with no upper age limit.

So buckle up and go for it. The Sky is the limit.

सर्वे भवन्तु सुखिनः । सर्वे सन्तु निरामयाः ।

सर्वे भद्राणि पश्यन्तु । मा कश्चिद् दुःख भाग् भवेत् ॥

ॐ शान्तिः शान्तिः शान्तिः ॥

When faith has blossomed in life, Every step is led by the Divine.

Sri Sri Ravi Shankar

Om Namah Shivaya जय गुरुदेव